HEALTH AND HUMAN DEVELOPMENT

PUBLIC HEALTH

IMPROVING HEALTH VIA INTER-PROFESSIONAL COLLABORATIONS

HEALTH AND HUMAN DEVELOPMENT

JOAV MERRICK - SERIES EDITOR –

NATIONAL INSTITUTE OF CHILD HEALTH AND HUMAN DEVELOPMENT,
MINISTRY OF SOCIAL AFFAIRS, JERUSALEM, ISRAEL

Adolescent Behavior Research: International Perspectives
Joav Merrick and Hatim A Omar (Editors)
2007. ISBN: 1-60021-649-8
(Hardcover)

Complementary Medicine Systems: Comparison and Integration
Karl W Kratky
2008. ISBN: 978-1-60456-475-4
(Hardcover)

Pain in Children and Youth
P Schofield and J Merrick (Editors)
2008. ISBN: 978-1-60456-951-3
(Hardcover)

Obesity and Adolescence: A Public Health Concern
Hatim A Omar, Donald E Greydanus, Dilip R Patel and Joav Merrick (Editors)
2009. ISBN: 978-1-60692-821-9
(Hardcover)

Poverty and Children: A Public Health Concern
Alexis Lieberman and Joav Merrick (Editors)
2009. ISBN: 978-1-60741-140-6
(Hardcover)

Living on the Edge: The Mythical, Spiritual, and Philosophical Roots of Social Marginality
Joseph Goodbread
2009. ISBN: 978-1-60741-162-8 (Hardcover)
2011. ISBN: 978-1-61470-192-7 (E-book)
2013. ISBN: 978-1-61122-986-8 (Softcover)

Social and Cultural Psychiatry Experience from the Caribbean Region
Hari D Maharajh and Joav Merrick (Editors)
2011. ISBN: 978-1-61668-506-5
(Hardcover)

Challenges in Adolescent Health: An Australian Perspective
David Bennett, Susan Towns and Elizabeth Elliott and Joav Merrick (Editors)
2009. ISBN: 978-1-60741-616-6
(Hardcover)

Children and Pain
P Schofield and J Merrick (Editors)
2009. ISBN: 978-1-60876-020-6
(Hardcover)

Alcohol-Related Cognitive Disorders: Research and Clinical Perspectives
Leo Sher, Isack Kandel and Joav Merrick (Editors)
2009. ISBN: 978-1-60741-730-9
(Hardcover)

Bone and Brain Metastases: Advances in Research and Treatment
Arjun Sahgal, Edward Chow and Joav Merrick (Editors)
2010. ISBN: 978-1-61668-365-8
(Hardcover)

Chance Action and Therapy: The Playful Way of Changing
Uri Wernik
2010. ISBN: 978-1-60876-393-1
(Hardcover)

International Aspects of Child Abuse and Neglect
Howard Dubowitz and Joav Merrick (Editors)
2010. ISBN: 978-1-61122-049-0
(Softcover)

Behavioral Pediatrics, 3rd Edition
Donald E Greydanus, Dilip R Patel, Helen D Pratt and Joseph L Calles Jr. (Editors)
2011. ISBN: 978-1-60692-702-1
(Hardcover)

Advances in Environmental Health Effects of Toxigenic Mold and Mycotoxins
Ebere Cyril Anyanwu
2011. ISBN: 978-1-60741-953-2
(Hardcover)

Rural Child Health: International Aspects
Erica Bell and Joav Merrick (Editors)
2011. ISBN: 978-1-60876-357-3
(Hardcover)

Principles of Holistic Psychiatry: A Textbook on Holistic Medicine for Mental Disorders
Soren Ventegodt and Joav Merrick
2011. ISBN: 978-1-61761-940-3
(Hardcover)

International Aspects of Child Abuse and Neglect
Howard Dubowitz and Joav Merrick (Editors)
2011. ISBN: 978-1-60876-703-8
(Hardcover)

Positive Youth Development: Evaluation and Future Directions in a Chinese Context
Daniel TL Shek, Hing Keung Ma and Joav Merrick (Editors)
2011. ISBN: 978-1-60876-830-1
(Hardcover)

Alternative Medicine Yearbook 2009
Joav Merrick (Editor)
2011. ISBN: 978-1-61668-910-0
(Hardcover)

Understanding Eating Disorders: Integrating Culture, Psychology and Biology
Yael Latzer, Joav Merrick and Daniel Stein (Editors)
2011. ISBN: 978-1-61728-298-0
(Hardcover)

Advanced Cancer, Pain and Quality of Life
Edward Chow and Joav Merrick (Editors)
2011. ISBN: 978-1-61668-207-1
(Hardcover)

Positive Youth Development: Implementation of a Youth Program in a Chinese Context
Daniel TL Shek, Hing Keung Ma and Joav Merrick (Editors)
2011. ISBN: 978-1-61668-230-9
(Hardcover)

Environment, Mood Disorders and Suicide
Teodor T Postolache and Joav Merrick (Editors)
2011. ISBN: 978-1-61668-505-8
(Hardcover)

Chance Action and Therapy: The Playful Way of Changing
Uri Wernik
2011. ISBN: 978-1-61122-987-5
(Softcover)

Public Health Yearbook 2009
Joav Merrick (Editor)
2011. ISBN: 978-1-61668-911-7
(Hardcover)

Child Health and Human Development Yearbook 2009
Joav Merrick (Editor)
2011. ISBN: 978-1-61668-912-4
(Hardcover)

Narratives and Meanings of Migration
Julia Mirsky
2011. ISBN: 978-1-61761-103-2
(Hardcover)

Self-Management and the Health Care Consumer
Peter William Harvey
2011. ISBN: 978-1-61761-796-6
(Hardcover)

Sexology from a Holistic Point of View
Soren Ventegodt and Joav Merrick
2011. ISBN: 978-1-61761-859-8
(Hardcover)

Clinical Aspects of Psychopharmacology in Childhood and Adolescence
DE Greydanus, JL Calles Jr, DP Patel, A Nazeer and J Merrick (Editors)
2011. ISBN: 978-1-61122-135-0
(Hardcover)

Drug Abuse in Hong Kong: Development and Evaluation of a Prevention Program
Daniel TL Shek, Rachel CF Sun and Joav Merrick (Editors)
2011. ISBN: 978-1-61324-491-3
(Hardcover)

Climate Change and Rural Child Health
Erica Bell, Bastian M Seidel and Joav Merrick (Editors)
2011. ISBN: 978-1-61122-640-9
(Hardcover)

Rural Medical Education: Practical Strategies
Erica Bell and Craig Zimitat and Joav Merrick (Editors)
2011. ISBN: 978-1-61122-649-2
(Hardcover)

Understanding Eating Disorders: Integrating Culture, Psychology and Biology
Yael Latzer, Joav Merrick and Daniel Stein (Editors)
2011. ISBN: 978-1-61470-976-3
(Softcover)

Positive Youth Development: Evaluation and Future Directions in a Chinese Context
Daniel TL Shek, Hing Keung Ma and Joav Merrick (Editors)
2011. ISBN: 978-1-62100-175-1
(Softcover)

The Dance of Sleeping and Eating among Adolescents: Normal and Pathological Perspectives
Yael Latzer and Orna Tzischinsky (Editors)
2011. ISBN: 978-1-61209-710-7
(Hardcover)

Randomized Clinical Trials and Placebo: Can You Trust the Drugs Are Working and Safe?
Søren Ventegodt and Joav Merrick
2011. ISBN: 978-1-61470-151-4 (E-book)
2012. ISBN: 978-1-61470-067-8 (Hardcover)

Child and Adolescent Health Yearbook 2009
Joav Merrick (Editor)
2012. ISBN: 978-1-61668-913-1
(Hardcover)

Applied Public Health: Examining Multifaceted Social or Ecological Problems and Child Maltreatment
John R Lutzker and Joav Merrick (Editors)
2012. ISBN: 978-1-62081-356-0 (Hardcover)

Adolescence and Chronic Illness. A Public Health Concern
Hatim Omar, Donald E Greydanus, Dilip R Patel and Joav Merrick (Editors)
2012. ISBN: 978-1-60876-628-4 (Hardcover)

Translational Research for Primary Healthcare
Erica Bell, Gert P Westert and Joav Merrick (Editors)
2012. ISBN: 978-1-61324-647-4 (Hardcover)

Child and Adolescent Health Yearbook 2010
Joav Merrick (Editor)
2012. ISBN: 978-1-61209-788-6 (Hardcover)

Child Health and Human Development Yearbook 2010
Joav Merrick (Editor)
2012. ISBN: 978-1-61209-789-3 (Hardcover)

Public Health Yearbook 2010
Joav Merrick (Editor)
2012. ISBN: 978-1-61209-971-2 (Hardcover)

The Astonishing Brain and Holistic Consciousness: Neuroscience and Vedanta Perspectives
Vinod D Deshmukh
2012. ISBN: 978-1-61324-295-7 (Hardcover)

Treatment and Recovery of Eating Disorders
Daniel Stein and Yael Latzer (Editors)
2012. ISBN: 978-1-61470-259-7 (Hardcover)
2013. ISBN: 978-1-62808-248-7 (Softcover)

Alternative Medicine Yearbook 2010
Joav Merrick (Editor)
2012. ISBN: 978-1-62100-132-4 (Hardcover)

Building Community Capacity: Minority and Immigrant Populations
Rosemary M Caron and Joav Merrick (Editors)
2012. ISBN: 978-1-62081-022-4 (Hardcover)

Human Immunodeficiency Virus (HIV) Research: Social Science Aspects
Hugh Klein and Joav Merrick (Editors)
2012. ISBN: 978-1-62081-293-8 (Hardcover)

AIDS and Tuberculosis: Public Health Aspects
Daniel Chemtob and Joav Merrick (Editors)
2012. ISBN: 978-1-62081-382-9 (Softcover)

Public Health Yearbook 2011
Joav Merrick (Editor)
2012. ISBN: 978-1-62081-433-8 (Hardcover)

Alternative Medicine Research Yearbook 2011
Joav Merrick (Editor)
2012. ISBN: 978-1-62081-476-5 (Hardcover)

Textbook on Evidence-Based Holistic Mind-Body Medicine: Basic Principles of Healing in Traditional Hippocratic Medicine
Søren Ventegodt and Joav Merrick
2012. ISBN: 978-1-62257-094-2 (Hardcover)

Textbook on Evidence-Based Holistic Mind-Body Medicine: Holistic Practice of Traditional Hippocratic Medicine
Søren Ventegodt and Joav Merrick
2012. ISBN: 978-1-62257-105-5
(Hardcover)

Textbook on Evidence-Based Holistic Mind-Body Medicine: Healing the Mind in Traditional Hippocratic Medicine
Søren Ventegodt and Joav Merrick
2012. ISBN: 978-1-62257-112-3
(Hardcover)

Textbook on Evidence-Based Holistic Mind-Body Medicine: Sexology and Traditional Hippocratic Medicine
Søren Ventegodt and Joav Merrick
2012. ISBN: 978-1-62257-130-7
(Hardcover)

Textbook on Evidence-Based Holistic Mind-Body Medicine: Research, Philosophy, Economy and Politics of Traditional Hippocratic Medicine
Søren Ventegodt and Joav Merrick
2012. ISBN: 978-1-62257-140-6
(Hardcover)

Building Community Capacity: Skills and Principles
Rosemary M Caron and Joav Merrick (Editors)
2012. ISBN 978-1-61209-331-4
(Hardcover)

Our Search for Meaning in Life: Quality of Life Philosophy
Soren Ventegodt and Joav Merrick
2012. ISBN: 978-1-61470-494-2
(Hardcover)

Health and Happiness from Meaningful Work: Research in Quality of Working Life
Soren Ventegodt and Joav Merrick (Editors)
2013. ISBN: 978-1-60692-820-2
(Hardcover)

Pediatric and Adolescent Sexuality and Gynecology: Principles for the Primary Care Clinician
Hatim A Omar, Donald E Greydanus, Artemis K Tsitsika, Dilip R Patel and Joav Merrick (Editors)
2013. ISBN: 978-1-60876-735-9
(Softcover)

Conceptualizing Behavior in Health and Social Research: A Practical Guide to Data Analysis
Said Shahtahmasebi and Damon Berridge
2013. ISBN: 978-1-60876-383-2
(Hardcover)

Adolescence and Sports
Dilip R Patel, Donald E Greydanus, Hatim Omar and Joav Merrick (Editors)
2013. ISBN: 978-1-60876-702-1
(Hardcover)

Human Development: Biology from a Holistic Point of View
Søren Ventegodt, Tyge Dahl Hermansen and Joav Merrick (Editors)
2013. ISBN: 978-1-61470-441-6
(Hardcover)

Building Community Capacity: Case Examples from Around the World
Rosemary M Caron and Joav Merrick (Editors)
2013. ISBN: 978-1-62417-175-8
(Hardcover)

Managed Care in a Public Setting
Richard Evan Steele
2013. ISBN: 978-1-62417-970-9
(Hardcover)

Alternative Medicine Research Yearbook 2012
Søren Ventegodt and Joav Merrick (Editors)
2013. ISBN: 978-1-62808-080-3
(Hardcover)

Health Promotion: Community Singing as a Vehicle to Promote Health
Joav Merrick (Editors)
2013. ISBN: 978-1-62618-908-9
(Softcover)

Public Health Yearbook 2012
Joav Merrick (Editor)
2013. ISBN: 978-1-62808-078-0
(Hardcover)

Health Risk Communication
Marijke Lemal and Joav Merrick (Editors)
2013. ISBN: 978-1-62257-544-2
(Hardcover)

Bullying: A Public Health Concern
Jorge C Srabstein and Joav Merrick (Editors)
2013. ISBN: 978-1-62618-564-7
(Hardcover)

Advanced Cancer: Managing Symptoms and Quality of Life
Natalie Pulenzas, Breanne Lechner, Nemica Thavarajah, Edward Chow and Joav Merrick (Editors)
2013. ISBN: 978-1-62808-239-5
(Hardcover)

Health Promotion: Strengthening Positive Health and Preventing Disease
Jing Sun, Nicholas Buys and Joav Merrick (Editors)
2013. ISBN: 978-1-62257-870-2
(Hardcover)

Pain Management Yearbook 2011
Joav Merrick (Editor)
2013. ISBN: 978-1-62808-970-7
(Hardcover)

Pain Management Yearbook 2012
Joav Merrick (Editor)
2013. ISBN: 978-1-62808-973-8
(Hardcover)

Food, Nutrition and Eating Behavior
Joav Merrick and Sigal Israeli
2013. ISBN: 978-1-62948-233-0
(Hardcover)

Public Health Concern: Smoking, Alcohol and Substance Use
Joav Merrick and Ariel Tenenbaum (Editors)
2013. ISBN: 978-1-62948-424-2
(Hardcover)

Mental Health from an International Perspective
Joav Merrick, Shoshana Aspler and Mohammed Morad (Editors)
2013. ISBN: 978-1-62948-519-5
(Hardcover)

Suicide from a Public Health Perspective
Said Shahtahmasebi and Joav Merrick
2014. ISBN: 978-1-62948-536-2
(Hardcover)

India: Health and Human Development Aspects
Joav Merrick (Editor)
2014. ISBN: 978-1-62948-784-7
(Hardcover)

Alternative Medicine Research Yearbook 2013
Joav Merrick (Editor)
2014. ISBN: 978-1-63321-094-3
(Hardcover)

Public Health Yearbook 2013
Joav Merrick (Editor)
2014. ISBN: 978-1-63321-095-0
(Hardcover)

Public Health: Improving Health via Inter-Professional Collaborations
Rosemary M. Caron and Joav Merrick (Editors)
2014. ISBN: 978-1-63321-569-6
(Hardcover)

HEALTH AND HUMAN DEVELOPMENT

PUBLIC HEALTH

IMPROVING HEALTH VIA INTER-PROFESSIONAL COLLABORATIONS

ROSEMARY M. CARON
AND
JOAV MERRICK
EDITORS

NOVA BIOMEDICAL

New York

For permission to use material from this book please contact us:
Telephone 631-231-7269; Fax 631-231-8175
Web Site: http://www.novapublishers.com

Library of Congress Cataloging-in-Publication Data

ISBN: 978-1-63321-569-6

Library of Congress Control Number: 2014945322

Published by Nova Science Publishers, Inc. † New York

Contents

Introduction

In: Public Health
Editors: Rosemary M. Caron and Joav Merrick

ISBN: 978-1-63321-569-6

Chapter 1

Public health: Improving health via inter-professional collaborations

Rosemary M Caron**, PhD, MPH*[1] *and
Joav Merrick, MD, MMedSc, DMSc[2,3,4,5,6]

[1] Department of Health Management and Policy, College of Health and Human Services, University of New Hampshire, Durham, New Hampshire, United States
[2] National Institute of Child Health and Human Development, Jerusalem
[3] Office of the Medical Director, Health Services, Division for Intellectual and Developmental Disabilities, Ministry of Social Affairs and Social Services, Jerusalem
[4] Division of Pediatrics, Hadassah Hebrew University Medical Center, Mt Scopus Campus, Jerusalem, Israel
[5] Kentucky Children's Hospital, University of Kentucky College of Medicine, Lexington, Kentucky, United States
[6] Center for Healthy Development, School of Public Health, Georgia State University, Atlanta, United States of America

It is often stated that "it takes a village" to improve the health of a population. This proverb implies that it takes the work of many individuals, not necessarily from the same occupation or educational or social background, to achieve this goal. To improve the health of a population, a system comprised of educators, community leaders, public health and health care practitioners, researchers, faith-based leaders, municipal workers, and many others working, in diverse urban and/or rural communities, across the globe towards a common goal via evidence-based practice, policy development, education and health literacy initiatives, or a combination thereof, is required.

Inter-professional collaborations can be fruitful endeavors with respect to improving health at a population and/or individual level. However, if we examine these interdisciplinary

* *Correspondence:* Rosemary M Caron, PhD, MPH, University of New Hampshire, College of Health and Human Services, Department of Health Management and Policy, #319 Hewitt Hall, 4 Library Way, Durham, New Hampshire, United States. E-mail: Rosemary.Caron@unh.edu.

collaborations from a development standpoint, not every professional is trained to work with professionals from other disciplines. How do we prepare an inter-professional workforce capable of working collaboratively? The Inter-professional Education Collaborative (IPEC), comprised of the following professional organizations: Association of American Medical Colleges, American Association of Colleges of Nursing, American Association of Colleges of Osteopathic Medicine, American Association of Colleges of Pharmacy, American Dental Education Association, and the Association of Schools of Public Health, convened to develop core competencies for those engaged in inter-professional collaborative practice (1). The IPEC's (1) competency domains are as follows:

- Values/ethics for inter-professional practice via patient-centered care and an appreciation of cultural differences of the teams providing care;
- Roles/responsibilities of an inter-professional team should be designated via the health needs of the population or patient;
- Inter-professional communication should occur to achieve the public health mission of disease prevention and health promotion;
- Teams should conduct their work in a manner that is efficient, effective, and equitable.

Furthermore, the discussion of Inter-professional Education (IPE) reiterates for us one of the major messages highlighted in the Institute of Medicine's (2) report titled "The Future of Public Health", which recommended that academic institutions should develop relationships with practice-oriented public health agencies, so that students, our future workforce, would not only engage in learning the requisite body of public health knowledge but also have the opportunity to develop the required skills to practice public health in the "real world" environment that is interdisciplinary in its everyday operation. For example, academic institutions that partner with clinics and community health centers for prevention education can serve as an opportunity to utilize IPE.

In summary, the importance of inter-professional education and collaboration is best stated by the World Health Organization's report (3):

"Once students understand how to work inter-professionally, they are ready to enter the workplace as a member of the collaborative practice team. This is a key step in moving health systems from fragmentation to a position of strength. Inter-professional health-care teams understand how to optimize the skills of their members, share case management and provide better health-services to patients and the community. The resulting strengthened health system leads to improved health outcomes."

We would also add that such an approach can contribute to achieving a healthier population at a reduced cost and in a more efficient manner. Inter-professional education and collaboration should be part of the cornerstones for improving a community's overall health status – the evidence-based research in this area supports this claim.

References

[1] Inter-professional Education Collaborative Expert Panel. Core competencies for inter-professional collaborative practice: Report of an expert panel. Washington, DC: Inter-professional Education Collaborative, 2011.

[2] Institute of Medicine. The Future of Public Health. Washington, DC: National Academy Press, 1988.

[3] World Health Organization. Framework for action on inter-professional education and collaborative practice, 2010. URL: http://www.who.int/hrh/resources/framework_action /en/index.html

Section one:
Inter-professional education

In: Public Health
Editors: Rosemary M. Caron and Joav Merrick
ISBN: 978-1-63321-569-6

Chapter 2

Innovations in continuing professional education to foster effective inter-professional collaboration

Linda J Mast[1*], Ateequr Rahman[2], Bard I Schatzman[1], Diane Bridges[1] and Neil Horsley[3]

[1]College of Health Professions, Rosalind Franklin University of Medicine and Science, North Chicago,
[2]College of Pharmacy, Rosalind Franklin University of Medicine and Science, North Chicago,
[3]Scholl College of Podiatric Medicine, Rosalind Franklin University of Medicine and Science, North Chicago, Illinois, US

This study addresses the critical need for innovation in public health workforce training and continuing education to foster effective inter-professional collaboration. The focus of this study was to assess the impact of inter-professional collaboration on practitioners who were charged with creating an inter-professional (IP) care model emphasizing primary and secondary prevention services specific for seniors with diabetes. The impact of inter-professional collaboration as an intervention for practitioners was assessed using a half day problem-based learning workshop and facilitated group sessions over a six month time period. Practitioner subjects representing disciplines of physicians assistant, physical therapy, pharmacy, nursing, registered dietician, and podiatry all participated in the intervention. Using an authentic task-based curriculum and guidelines for required care protocols, these practitioner subjects completed a specific workshop about IP care collaboration and four facilitated work sessions. The impact of participating in an IP team was measured using pre-test and post-test instruments including the Inter-professional Education Perception Scale (IEPS) to assess attitudes and the Concerns Based Adoption Model (C-BAM) to assess actual behaviors related to inter-professional collaboration. Results of this research provided a workforce training and facilitated team building model that can be used to enhance inter-professional collaboration. The study demonstrates a

* Corresponding author: Linda J. Mast, PhD, Rosalind Franklin University of Medicine and Science, 3333 Green Bay Road, North Chicago, IL 60064, United States. E-mail: linda.mast@rosalindfranklin.edu.

process for implementing a continuing education program that engages an inter-professional healthcare team in the creation of an effective preventive care model. This preventive care model responds to the need to develop new methods for ongoing training of the public health workforce in an inter-professional collaborative process. Initial findings are promising in that this innovative approach to continuing education resulted in both increased inter-professional collaboration behaviors and more favorable attitudes about working in inter-professional teams.

Introduction

Challenges exist for public health workforce development in both developing countries and wealthier countries alike. Beaglehole and Dal Poz (1) relate this challenge to the traditional emphasis on formal academic and didactic training with very limited attention being paid to training methods that are field-based continuing education where the workforce can participate in work group training that addresses the diversity and complexity of the healthcare team from a wide range of occupational backgrounds (1). Patients today have complex medical issues requiring more than one healthcare professional which calls for inter-professional collaboration (2). In 2001, acknowledging the medically challenging needs of patients, the Institute of Medicine (IOM) Committee on Quality of Health Care in America recommended that healthcare professionals be able to work in inter-professional (IP) teams (3). The research of Schofield et al. demonstrated that, especially for complex, chronic conditions, a multidisciplinary, or IP, team offers many advantages for patients and their families (4). Bringing an inter-professional focus to the development of innovative care delivery models requires collaboration among the health professions to increase learning about, from and with each other, as well as incorporation of a patient centered perspective (5). A growing consensus exists that inter-professional (IP) team- based care offers the potential to improve quality of care and lower costs (6). However, Varda et al. emphasize that even though there is growing interest in collaborative practice in public health, there is still little empirical evidence within the public health literature to support and inform this practice (7). According to Gebbie and Turnock, public health is especially challenged due to the multidisciplinary nature of services provided (8), and there is often very limited opportunities for workforce training and continuing education interventions that address the need for inter-professional collaboration. In November 2012 the Global Health Forum on Innovation in Health Professional Education convened in Washington, D.C. One of the obstacles identified for implementing IP education was “knowing how to weave IP content into meaningful clinical and community experiences” (9). Such obstacles, while challenging for students, become even more daunting when the learners are practicing clinicians where continuing education programs need to be relevant to current practice needs, and delivered in ways that encourage professional development. This study provides a model for continuing education that addresses the need to engage learners in ways that use authentic tasks to develop inter-professional collaboration.

Collaborative partnerships in practice

Bringing an inter-professional focus to the development of innovative care delivery models requires collaboration among the health professions to increase learning about, from and with each other (10), as well as incorporation of a patient centered perspective. Continuing professional education research emphasizes that educating working professionals must use authentic projects that have relevance in practice. To date, there is very limited research addressing knowledge translation or continuing professional education within the inter-professional context (11). Further, the World Health Organization (WHO) supports the development of evidence to inform best approaches to public health workforce development (1).

Inter-professional teams develop through inter-professional collaboration. Inter-professional collaboration is a "partnership between a team of health providers and a client in a participatory collaborative and coordinated approach to shared decision making around health and social issues" (12). These collaborations "create an inter-professional practice team where healthcare providers from different professional backgrounds work together with patients, families, and communities to deliver the best quality of care."(13).

Inter-professional collaborative practice encompasses the synergistic input of each individual team member's skill and knowledge through a process of effective communication and decision making (14). Blending of professional cultures, shared skills, respect, accountability, coordination, cooperation, mutual trust and autonomy are components of an inter-professional collaborative practice (13-15). According to Bromage (16), this approach to team working, known as inter-professionalism, emphasizes highly collaborative problem-solving. This inter-professional team approach allows sharing of professional expertise with the ultimate goal of improving patient outcomes while sharing resources. (2,5). The intent of inter-professional teams is to collaborate and communicate closely with other healthcare professionals to achieve this common goal (17). However, U.S. public health workforce enumeration data suggests only 20% of the workforce had the education and training needed to work most effectively, and, therefore, a continuing education model that supports close integration of all health personnel is needed (18).

Continuing professional education (CPE) for inter-professional collaboration

The field of inter-professional education has been growing, and in May of 2011, an inter-professional panel representing the professions of allopathic medicine (AAMC), pharmacy (AACP), nursing (AANA), osteopathic medicine (AACOM), and dentistry (ADEA) established four domains for inter-professional competencies designed to guide the educational process for healthcare professionals: 1) Values/Ethics; 2) Roles/Responsibilities; 3) Inter-professional Communication; 4) Teams/teamwork (19). Although strides have been made to advance inter-professional care across the professions, there are still significant gaps between current needs for enhanced inter-professional collaboration and what is in practice in primary and preventive services (20).

Challenges exist for new graduates entering into professional practice where strong territorial cultures and barriers to inter-professional collaboration (i.e., silos) persist (19). This means that recent graduates may be prepared to engage in IP collaboration, but then find themselves immersed in healthcare delivery cultures that have not kept pace with advances in IP models of care. There are powerful influences of professional enculturation and limited understanding of continuing professional education (CPE) and actual change in practice (21). IP collaboration must include inter-professional education, inter-professional practice and inter-professional interventions (22). Continuing education that includes inter-professional education is critical in order to prepare practicing professionals to effectively collaborate. The Institute of Medicine (IOM) Committee on Planning a Continuing Health Care Professional Education Institute completed an in depth study of continuing education for the health professions that concluded team-based health care delivery is necessary, and that effective continuing education for healthcare professionals will be grounded in ways to engage practitioners in authentic work that has patient care and population health as its focus (9).

Consequently, for this study, the Problem-based learning (PBL) model was selected for a half-day workshop because it was determined that PBL would be an ideal approach to use as a way to assess impact on inter-professional collaboration attitudes and behaviors within the context of an authentic problem and work setting.

Problem based learning model for CPE

Problem based learning (PBL) originated as a teaching strategy at McMaster University in the 1960s and has since been adopted throughout North America and worldwide (23). Barrows (24) developed a taxonomy of PBL types to better define the key elements of this educational format. It is generally characterized as an instructional method where small groups of learners address a specific patient problem. The PBL approach was selected as the instructional method (the intervention) for the CPE workshop because it engages participants in a small group environment and is grounded in authentic problem solving tasks. This is supported by the theoretical foundation that adult learners prefer the use of authentic practice settings that include a problem to be solved. (25–26). PBL has been used in prior inter-professional continuing education programs where participants learned about the roles and contributions of other health professions within the context of an authentic task (26).

Continuing professional education (CPE) instructional design

This study used a PBL half day workshop and facilitated follow up group meetings led by a professional group facilitator to encourage inter-professional collaboration within the context of developing a preventive care model for older adults with Type 2 diabetes. The workshop included an authentic case study to engage the participants in an inter-professional discussion to model the expectations of PBL work. This was followed by introduction of the assigned task to develop a care model to provide primary and secondary preventive services to seniors with diabetes. Details of the instructional design for the program are provided in table 1.

Table 1. Workshop Instructional Design

Workshop Curriculum				
Introductions and Welcome	Research Team and Participant Introductions	Welcome greetings from a recognized leader in Inter-professional education	Overview of workshop materials (includes strategically selected journal articles on IP collaboration and diabetes that were pre-selected by the researchers to give participants some foundational research sources)	Pre test surveys completed
Group Activity to Introduce the Problem Based Learning Process	Initial group work (non directed) to engage participants in working together	Tour of facilities where care will be provided (ambulatory care clinic and a mobile care unit)	Time for relationship building among practitioner subjects	Discovery and discussion based on workshop materials and journal articles
Experiential Case relevant to benefits of IP collaboration (Specific to Diabetes and Community Needs)	Authentic case presented on a senior with diabetes	Participant subjects discuss what they identify as top priorities	Discussion on how top priorities may vary based on practitioner discipline.	Discovery and discussion on value of IP collaboration.
Authentic Task Introduction and Assignment	IP participants introduced to the authentic task to develop an IP care model for seniors with diabetes based on primary and secondary prevention	Timeline for completion and parameters of the objective are discussed	IP participants are asked to identify and appoint a group leader for their PBL team and team process	Care model is implemented at clinical location sites
Follow up collaborative sessions with guided reflection worksheets and facilitator	Participant group leader (PBL team leader) continues collaborative meetings with participants to begin developing the care model.	Professional Group facilitator coordinates follow up meetings with PBL team leader for month 3 and 6 of the six month process	Debriefing session with participant PBL team, professional group facilitator and research team.	Post-test surveys completed

The advantage of using the PBL curriculum design is that it focuses on team building and inquiry in the PBL context. This continuing education model can be customized to meet the needs of any specific community's health priorities, whether rural or urban, by selecting a focused and relevant case study that allows participants to work toward desired outcomes related to improved patient care.

Our study

The population for potential subjects was limited to clinical practitioners working in one healthcare organization. Written informed consent was obtained from each practitioner subject following Protocol IPHS #001 as approved by the authors' Institutional Review Board. A purposive sample was obtained to represent registered nurses, physical therapists, physicians, physician assistants, registered dieticians, pharmacists, and podiatrists (the physician did not complete the study due to geographic relocation). Practitioner subjects participated in a half day PBL based workshop followed by monthly facilitated discussions with the task of developing an IP care model for seniors with diabetes.

Intervention

The half-day workshop was designed to immerse participants in experiential learning about inter-professional concepts centered on the core inter-professional competencies (19). Application of these concepts used patient simulations, debriefing discussions and team based activities using a social learning framework that have been demonstrated to be effective for team building within a professional context (28-29). The content for the workshop was developed by faculty experts in group dynamics, leading changes, and delivery of CPE programs for health care professionals. The program was delivered in an interactive conference style setting, and the assigned task for the participants in the workshop was based on community needs assessment data from the local public health department. At the workshop, the practitioner subjects were assigned the task of creating a comprehensive, patient–centered care model for delivering prevention services for seniors with diabetes.

Participation in the process of creating the inter-professional care (IP) model served as the experiential lab for the study of the participants' IP collaboration experience. The follow up facilitated group meetings were based on inter-professional protocols established by Belanger and Rodriguez (30), including significant investment in time and training, clear role development, communication strategies, trust and respect, and systems to guide cooperative practice. Participants in the study were made aware that their newly created inter-professional care model for preventive services would be implemented and used over a six month time interval to evaluate patient outcomes and to measure any changes in inter-professional collaboration perspectives among clinician participants. The intervention process was sequenced as follows for practitioner participants:

1. Pre-implementation: Collection of pre-test Concerns-Based Adoption Model (CBAM) Levels of Use (LoU) and Inter-professional Education Perception Scale (IEPS) data.
2. Half day workshop: Program introduced foundation information about the target patient population, the mobile care unit facility and inter-professional collaboration. The workshop was designed as an integrated process; the teams were supported by inter-professional faculty and by specialists in inter-professional education.

   An overview of expectations of the project was provided. Content included experiential activities and the focus will be on team building and the four established competencies of inter-professional collaboration.

3. IP Care Model development: The practitioner subjects completed four self-directed PBL sessions of 1-2 hours to develop the inter-professional care model to be implemented for older adult patients with Type 2 diabetes. The CPE workshop content included specific guidelines for the care protocol process and established designation of assigned professionals to work with patients. Each member of the inter-professional team focused on the various aspects of the project as clinician, providing clinical care for patients as educator, and as innovator, contributing to the ongoing refinement and evaluation of the inter-professional practice model. Informal discussion and email exchanges among the team in smaller groups occurred routinely throughout the process. Goldman's work with IP group facilitation informed the design of four sessions as follows: a. Review objectives, examine clinical evidence with focus on primary and secondary prevention, explore barriers and enablers to change, needs assessment for assigned patient population; b. Review needs assessment using mind mapping to finalize an ideal delivery pathway and present to IP peers. Use evidence and literature support to support selected pathway; c. Draft inter-professional model care protocols; d. Refine protocol and organize materials to implement the IP care model (22).
4. Debriefings: Six monthly inter-professional debriefings were completed. Four were conducted by the group leader chosen by the participant subjects and two, one at mid-point and at the end, were conducted by an expert group facilitator for thirty minutes to one hour to discuss the inter-professional care model delivery as it progresses. At the end, the team came together for a final debriefing and discussion. During this time, review and assessment was done, which included a list of the issues identified and addressed as well as any outstanding concerns and a proposed management plan for these concerns.
5. Post-test data collection: Post test CBAM-LoU and IEPS data were collected at the end of the six month IP care model intervention.

Research questions

This research project addressed the following research questions pertaining to clinical practitioner subjects:

1. Are there differences among clinical professionals' behaviors related to inter-professional collaboration?
2. Are there differences among clinical professionals' perceptions of inter-professional collaboration?
3. Does participation in an inter-professional care team impact clinical professionals' perceptions and behaviors with regard to inter-professional collaboration?

Dependent variables

Two instruments were used to collect pre test and post test data. These were the Inter-professional Education Perception Scale (IEPS), and the Concerns-Based Adoption Model-Level of Use (CBAM-LoU).

Dependent variable measures:

1. Total IEPS Scores
2. IEPS sub scores
3. CBAM-LoU scores
4. CBAM-LoU sub scores over 8 dimensions

Independent variable (practitioner):

1. Clinical profession

Measures

Data collection

The IEPS and CBAM-LoU instruments were used to collect pre- and post-test data related to attitudes about IP collaboration (IEPS) and behaviors related to IP collaboration. Pre-test data was collected at the workshop and facilitated meeting sites. Post-test data was collected at the end of the six month implementation of the IP care model.

The Interdisciplinary Education Perception Scale (IEPS)

The Interdisciplinary Education Perception Scale (IEPS) was developed by Luecht et al. (31) and has been widely used to assess attitudes about inter-professional education among graduate and undergraduate students. In this study, however, the instrument was used to assess the attitudes of professionals in practice. More recently, an alternative, remodeled twelve item instrument has been developed consolidating the four original subscales into three. The revised instrument (IEPS Model 7) with three subscales of Competency and Autonomy, Perceived Need for Cooperation, and Perception of Actual Cooperation was used for this study. Construct validity of the IEPS was confirmed in using expert feedback from interdisciplinary health care professionals for each survey item (32). The remodeled IEPS instrument is considered a stable and reliable instrument with good internal consistency of the total scale with Chronbach's alpha of 0.86 (32).

The Concerns-Based Adoption Model - Levels of Use (CBAM-LoU v1.1)

The Concerns-Based Adoption Model - Levels of Use (CBAM-LoU v1.1) is a focused interview process that has been used to describe behaviors of those engaged in an innovation or change as they progress through levels of use. It does not focus on attitudinal, motivational, or other affective aspects of the user. The CBAM LoU interview process has been widely used in studies related to change and innovation. It is based on the eight levels of use defined as: (0) Non-Use, (I) Orientation, (II) Preparation, (III) Mechanical Use, (IVA) Routine, (IVB) Refinement, (V) Integration, and (VI) Renewal. It is an ideal instrument to measure changes over time along a continuum (34). Test-retest reliability and alpha of 0.84 – 0.87 has been demonstrated (33). It has been used in many published empirical studies over the past thirty years (35). Although it has been most frequently used in education, more recently it has been adapted for research in the department of defense and health care. A limitation of the CBAM-

LoU is the potential for variability in scoring among reviewers and the need for strict adherence to the focused interview protocols. In depth training for researchers conducting and scoring the focused interview ensures that scoring results are based on the prescribed process following decision points from the subject's responses.

Results

Participant subjects included one registered nurse, one physician assistant, one psychiatrist (who did not complete participation due to relocation to another state), one pharmacist, one podiatrist, and one physical therapist.

Scoring

IEPS

The IEPS is a twelve item self report survey instrument. Each of the seven practitioner subjects were asked to indicate their level of agreement with each statement using a six point Likert type scale (6= Strongly Agree; 5= Agree; 4= Somewhat Agree; 2= Disagree; 1= Strongly Disagree). The IEPS was completed prior to the half day workshop as a pre-test, and again as a post-test at the completion of the six months of facilitated group meetings that followed the workshop.

For each sub-scale (SS1, SS2, SS3) items are grouped based on a specific construct related to inter-professional team work. Highest possible scores are shown in Table 2.

CBAM-LoU

The CBAM-LoU is an interview based assessment that assesses actual behaviors related to an innovation. For this study IP collaboration was the innovation introduced to the subjects during the pre-test and post-test private interviews. Pre-test interview results indicated that most subjects had limited or mechanical use of IP collaboration. Post-test interviews at the end of the six months of the study revealed positive trends with IP collaboration behaviors for all subjects. Some subjects behaviors related to IP collaboration advanced to refinement and integration in to their practice. Table 3 highlights results of the pre-test and post-test CBAM-LoU interviews.

Table 2. IEPS Highest Possible Scores (Total and Sub-scales)

Scale Section	Highest Possible Score
Total score	72
SS1	30
SS2	12
SS3	30

Table 3. Subject Ratings of Levels of Use (of Inter-professional Collaboration)

Subject#	Pretest	Posttest
1	II	IVa
2	III	IV a
3	I	III
4	II	VI
5	IVa	V
6	III	IVa

Results of private interviews with a member of the research team who was trained in the CBAM-LoU interview protocol were rated by four members of the research team to ensure consistent results with ratings for levels of use. The interview process is based on a very structured and truncated interview style designed to provide consistent results as illustrated in figure 1.

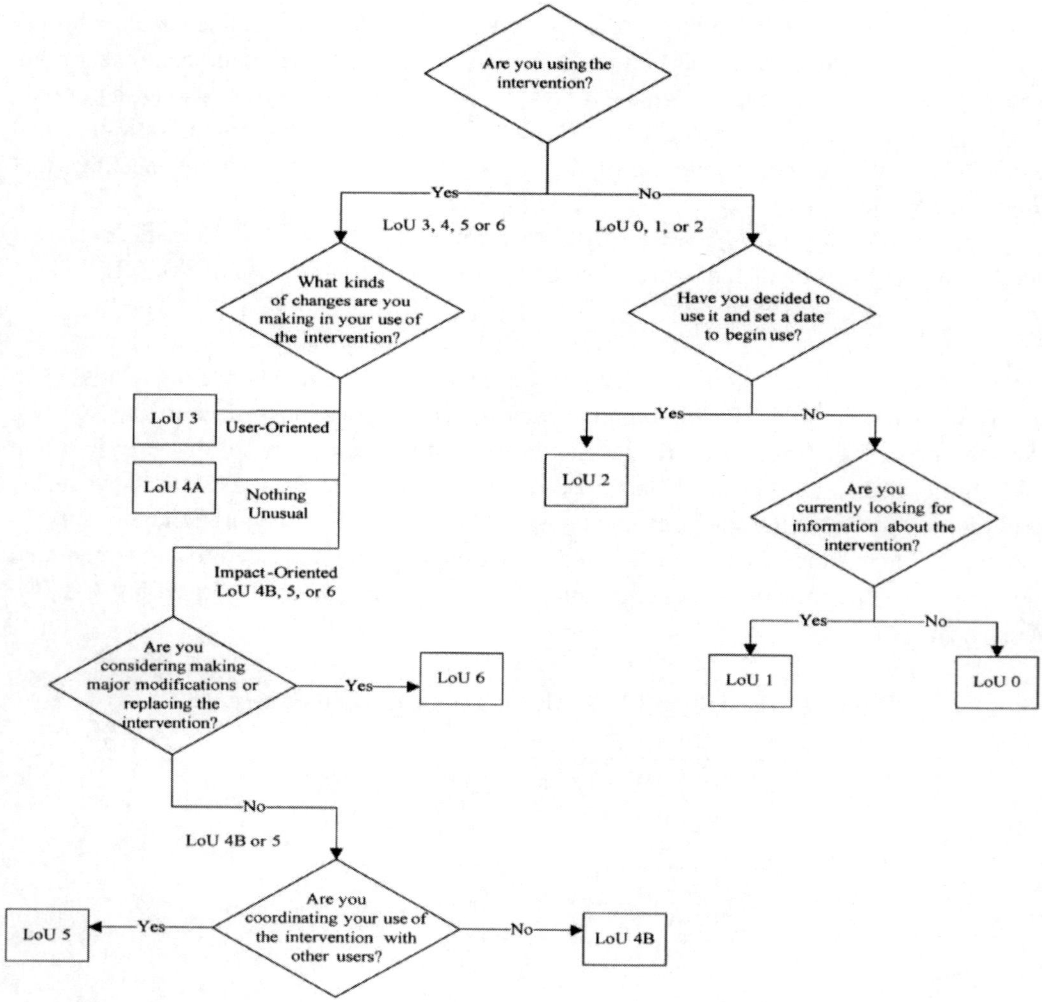

Figure 1. CBAM-LoU Branching Chart (36).

Table 4. Levels of Use of the Innovation (36)

0	*Nonuse:* State in which user has little or no knowledge of the innovation.
I	*Orientation*: State in which the user has acquired or is acquiring information about the innovation, and is exploring its value.
II	*Preparation:* State in which the user is preparing for first use of the innovation.
III	*Mechanical Use:* State in which the user focuses most effort on the short-term day to day use of the innovation with little time for reflection.
IVA	*Routine:* Use of the innovation is stabilized. Few if any changes are being made in the ongoing use. Little preparation or thought is being given to improving the innovation.
IVB	*Refinement:* State in which the user varies the use of the innovation to increase the impact on clients within immediate sphere of influence.
V	*Integration:* State in which the user is combining own efforts to use the innovation with the related activities of colleagues to achieve a collective effect on clients within their common sphere of influence.
VI	*Renewal:* State in which the user reevaluates the quality of the use of the innovation, seeks major modifications or alternatives to the present innovation to achieve increased impact on clients.

Levels of use are a behavioral phenomenon that does not address attitudes or feelings. It only addresses what subjects actually do. For this reason, it was an ideal companion to the IEPS survey that measures only attitudes in order to get a broader understanding of both attitudes and behaviors regarding IP collaboration. Levels of use include eight levels that range from nonuse to renewal as outlined in table 4.

Analysis

IEPS

The IEPS survey instrument assesses self-reported attitudes regarding IP collaboration. Using the remodeled instrument (39), total IEPS scores and the three sub-scores were compared across practitioners for differences between professions, as well as to identify changes in scores that may have occurred over time based on the six months of facilitated collaboration following the PBL workshop. Total IEPS scores and the three sub-scores were compared across professions, prior to the workshop and following the workshop and six months of facilitated collaboration. See Table 5 for descriptive statistics.

Table 5. IEPS Descriptive Statistics

Practitioner Subject	Total Score (Pre-test)	SS1	SS2	SS3	Total Score (Post-test)	SS1	SS2	SS3
1	58	24	11	23	57	24	10	23
2	66	27	11	28	66	27	10	29
3	58	24	10	24	65	28	12	25
4	22	7	3	12	64	26	11	27
5	61	26	9	26	66	28	12	26
6	50	22	11	17	63	26	11	26
7	Did not complete the study				Did not complete the study			
MEAN SCORES	52.5	21.7	9.2	21.7	63.5	26.5	11	26

n=6.

Table 6. Comparison of Mean Pre-test & Post-test Scores

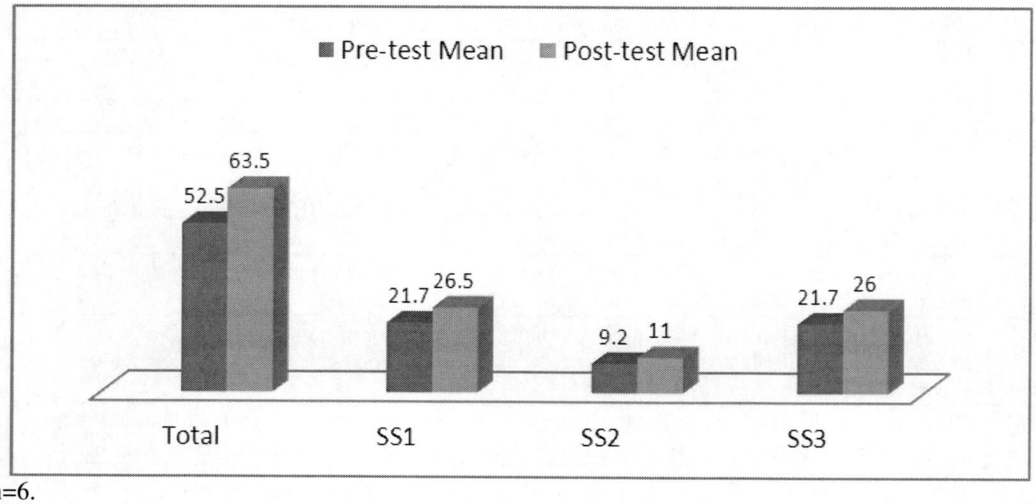

n=6.

Total scores ranged from 22 to 66 with a mean score of 52.5. Notably the lowest score came from a subject with no prior knowledge or experience with IP collaboration. Other participants all had prior knowledge and experience with IP. Based on pre-test and post-test scores, consistent positive trends in both total scores and all sub scores were observed. See Table 6.

Comparison of pre-test and post test scores for each individual participant also resulted in positive trend with increased total scores and increases for all sub scores. Notably, the subject with no prior knowledge or experience had post test scores in similar ranges with other subjects who came to the study with prior IP knowledge and experience. See tables 7- 10.

Table 7. Total Scores by Subject (Practitioners)

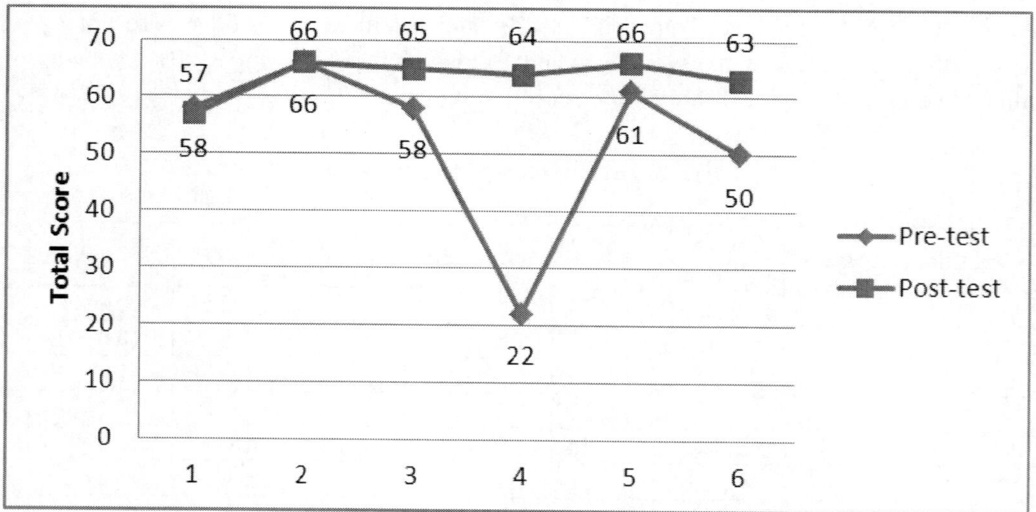

n=6.

Table 8. Comparison of Mean Pre-test & Post-test SS1 Scores

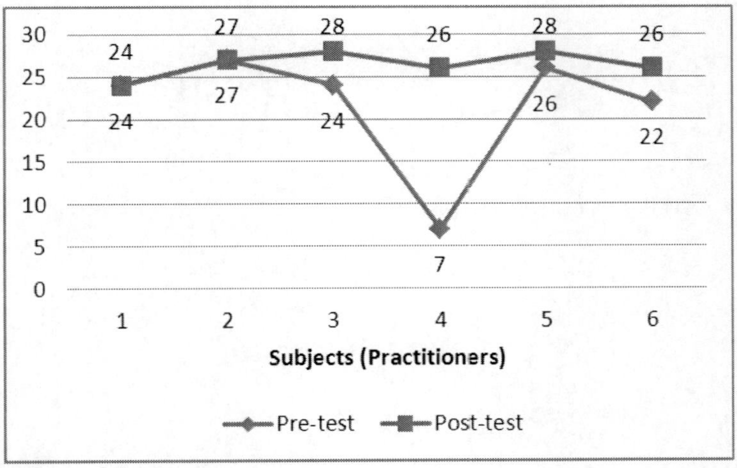

n=6 SS1 Competency and Autonomy.

Table 9. Comparison of Mean Pre-test & Post-test SS2 Scores

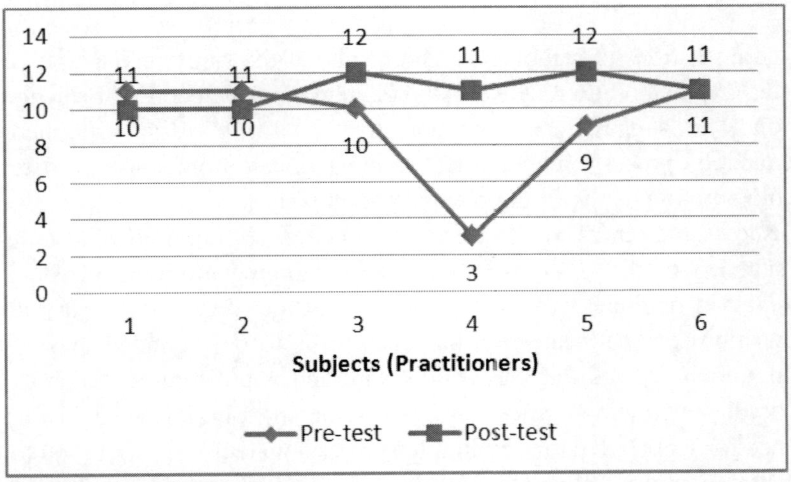

n=6 SS2 Perceived Need for Cooperation.

CBAM-LoU

The pre-test results of the CBAM-LoU interviews indicated most subjects were at the Orientation or Preparation level of use. One individual was at Mechanical Use and one was at Routine level. The subject who was at Orientation level was the subject with no prior inter-professional experience and the subject at Routine level had the most prior experience and had worked previously at an organization that promoted inter-professional collaboration. Post- test results indicated positive trends with increased inter-professional collaboration behaviors. The subject with no prior experience increased from Orientation to Mechanical Use, and all other subjects were at either Routine levels of use or Integration.

Table 10. Comparison of Mean Pre-test 7 Post-test SS3 Scores

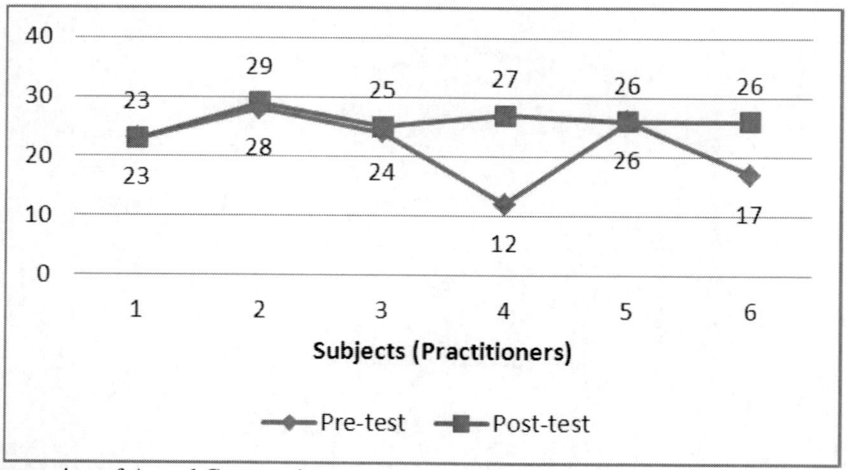

n=6 SS3 Perception of Actual Cooperation.

Discussion

Recognizing the limitations of sample size, the results of the study indicate positive changes in attitude about IP collaboration, as well as moderate enhancements in behaviors regarding IP collaboration. This suggests there are potential benefits of using a defined continuing professional education process, such as PBL, to create an environment that fosters the inter-professional collaboration that will improve patient outcomes.

Evidence shows that there are powerful influences of professional enculturation and limited understanding of the relationship between continuing professional education (CPE) and actual change in practice. Team-based health care delivery is necessary and effective continuing education for healthcare professionals needs to be grounded in ways to engage practitioners in authentic work that has patient care and population health as its focus. The PBL model for the continuing professional education intervention used in this study can provide guidance for workforce training in inter-professional (IP) collaboration to develop IP care models that may improve clinical outcomes and care delivery efficiencies.

This study addresses the critical need for innovation in workforce training and professional development through continuing education. It demonstrates a process for implementing a PBL continuing education process that is grounded in adult learning theory and authentic task content. The results of this study give direction for future research with expanded populations of practitioners in public health settings.

Limitations for practitioner subject analysis are as follows: Due to the nature of the practitioner environment, totally randomized subjects will not be feasible. In addition, the research will not be able to control for dispositional factors of individual practitioners, and the relatively small sample size of practitioner subjects. Further, the one group pre-test, post- test design provides a measure of change but does not provide conclusive results about its cause.

Findings of this study may serve as a model for future research opportunities to implement this PBL based continuing educational model across larger groups of public health provider communities.

Acknowledgments

This study was financially supported by the Office of Sponsored Research at Rosalind Franklin University of Medicine and Science. The contributions of Kevin Morris and Rafeda Khan, who are both students in the Doctor of Pharmacy program in the College of Pharmacy at Rosalind Franklin University of Medicine and Science, were instrumental in the implementation of the CPE workshop. The researchers would also like to express appreciation to Gene Hall, PhD, Professor of Educational Leadership at the University of Nevada in Las Vegas for his guidance on use of the CBAM-Lou and to Richard Luecht, PhD, University of North Carolina at Greensboro. Professor and Chair of the Department of Educational Research Methodology and Director of the Center for Educational Research and Evaluation (CERE), for his generous permission to use the IEPS instrument.

References

[1] Beaglehole R, Dal Poz MR. Public Health workforce: Challenges and policy issues Hum Resour Health 2003;1(1):4.

[2] Lumague M, Morgan A, Mak D, Hanna M, Kwong J, Cameron C, Zener D, Sinclair L. Inter-professional education: The student perspective. J Interprof Care 2008;20(3):246-53.

[3] Institute of Medicine. Redesigning continuing education in the health professions. Washington, DC: National Academy Press, 2009.

[4] Schofield D, Fuller J, Wagner S, Friis L, Tyrell B. Multidisciplinary management of complex care. Aust J Rural Health 2009;17(1):45-48.

[5] Barker, K, & Oandasan I. Inter-professional care review with medical residents: Lessons learned, tensions aired-A pilot study. J Interprof Care 2005;19(3):207-14.

[6] Fisher E, Bynum J, Skinner J. The policy implications of variations in Medicare spending growth. 2009. Accessed 2012 Dec 2. URL: http://www.dartmouthatlas.org/downloads/reports/Policy_Implications_Brief_022709.pdf

[7] Varda D, Shoup J, Miller SA. Systematic review of collaboration and network research in the public affairs literature: Implications for public health practice and research. Amer J Public Health 2012;102(3):564-71.

[8] Gebbie KM, Turnock BJ. The public health workforce, 2006: New challenges. Health Aff 2006;25(4):923-33.

[9] IOM (Institute of Medicine). Inter-professional education for collaboration: Learning how to improve health from inter-professional models across the continuum of education to practice: Workshop summary. Washington, DC: The National Academies Press. 2013.

[10] Centre for the Advancement of Inter-professional Education (CAIPE). Accessed June 12, 2013. URL: http://caipe.org.uk/about-us/defining-ipe/

[11] Zwarenstein M, Reeves S. Knowledge translation and inter-professional collaboration: Where the rubber of evidence-based care hits the road of teamwork. J Contin Educ Health Prof 2006;26(1):46-54.

[12] Canadian Inter-professional Health Collaborative. A national inter-professional competency framework; February 2010. Accessed June 12, 2013. URL: http://www.cihc.ca/files/CIHC_IPCompetencies_ Feb1210.pdf.

[13] Freeth D, Hammick M, Reeves S, Koppel I, Barr H. Effective inter-professional education: Development, delivery and evaluation. Oxford: Blackwell, 2005.

[14] Kasperski M. Implementation strategies: Collaboration in primary care family doctors and nurse practitioners delivering shared care. Toronto, ON: Ontario College of Family Physicians, 2000. Accessed June 12, 2013. URL: http://www.cfpc.ca/English/CFPC/CLFM/bibnursing/default.asp?s_1.

[15] Morrison S. Working together: Why bother with collaboration? Work Based Learning in Primary Care 2007;5:65-70.

[16] Bromage A. Inter-professional education. higher education resources 2009. Accessed: September 15, 2011. URL: http://highereducationresources.atspace.com/inter-professional.htm

[17] Barr H, Koppel I, Reeves S, Hammick M, Freeth, D. Effective inter-professional education: Development, delivery and evaluation. Oxford: Blackwell, 2005.

[18] USA public health workforce enumeration. Accessed December 12, 2013. URL: http://bhpr.hrsa.gov/healthworkforce/reports/publichealthstudy2005.pdf.

[19] Schmitt M et al. Core competencies for inter-professional collaborative practice.The Inter-professional Education Collaborative (IPEC). Accessed December 12, 2013. URL: http://www.asph.org/userfiles/collaborativepractice.pdf.

[20] Young L, Baker P, Waller S, Hodgson L, Moor M. Knowing your allies: Medical education and inter-professional exposure. J Interprof Care 2007;21(2):155-63.

[21] Umble KE, Cervero RM, Langone CA. Negotiating about power frames, and continuing education: A case study in public health. Adult Educ Q 2001;51(2):128.

[22] Goldman J, Zwarenstein M, Bhattacharyya O, Reeves, S. Improving the clarity of the inter-professional field: implications for research and continuing inter-professional education. J Contin Educ Health Prof 2009;29(3):151-6.

[23] Albanese M, Mitchell S. Problem-based learning: A review of literature on its outcomes and implementation issues. Acad Med 1993;68(1):52-81.

[24] Barrows H. A taxonomy of problem-based learning methods. Med Educ 1986;20:481-86.

[25] Cervero RM, Wilson AL, Associates. Power in practice: Adult education and the struggle for knowledge and power in society. San Francisco: Jossey-Bass, 2001.

[26] Moore DE, Pennington FC. Practice-based learning and improvement. J Educ Health Prof 2003;23 (Spring Suppl- 1):S73-80.

[27] Mann K, Viscount P, Cogdon A, Davidson K, Langille D, MacCara M. Multidisciplinary learning in continuing professional education: The heart health Nova Scotia experience. J Contin Educ Health Prof 1996;16(1):135-41.

[28] Vygotsky LS. Mind in society: Development of higher psychological processes.(Cole M, John-Steiner V, Scribner S, Souberman E, eds.). Cambridge, MA: Harvard University Press, 1978.

[29] Bandura A. Self-efficacy: The exercise of control. New York: WH Freeman, 1997.

[30] Belanger E, Rodriguez C. More than the sum of its parts? A qualitative research synthesis on multi-disciplinary primary care teams. J Interprof Care 2008;22(6):587-97.

[31] Luecht R, Madsen M, Taugher M, Peterson B. Assessing professional perceptions: Design and validation of an interdisciplinary education principle scale. J Allied Health, 1990; 19(2): 181-6.

[32] McFadden AK, McLaren WM, Webster VS. The Interdisciplinary Education Perception Scale (IEPS): An alternative remodeled sub-scale structure and its Reliability. Strategies for implementing innovative clinical practices. J Interprof Care 2007;21(4):433-43.

[33] Khoboli B, O'Toole J. The concerns based adoption model: Teachers participation in action research. Syst Pract Action Res 2012;25(2):137-48.

[34] Hancock R, Knezek G, Christensen R. Cross validating measures of technology integration: A first step toward examining potential relationships between technology integration and student achievement. J Computing Teacher Educ 2007;24 (1):15-21.

[35] Hall G, Hord S. Implementing change: Patterns principles and potholes. Boston, MA: Pearson Education 2006.

[36] Hall G, Dirksen D, George A. Measures of Implementation in schools: Levels of use. Austin, TX: SEDL, 2006.

In: Public Health
Editors: Rosemary M. Caron and Joav Merrick

ISBN: 978-1-63321-569-6

Chapter 3

An interdisciplinary and inter-professional dual degree program for public health training in a new rural medical school

Mark V White*, MD, MPH[1], Olapeju M Simoyan, MD, MPH, BDS[1], Alberto JF Cardelle, PhD, MPH[2], Steven Godin, PhD, MPH[2], Elizabeth C Kuchinski, MPH[1], Erica L Townsend, BS[1] and Janet M Townsend, MD[1]

[1]Department of Family, Community, and Rural Health, The Commonwealth Medical College (TCMC), Scranton, Pennsylvania

[2]The College of Health Sciences, Department of Health Studies, East Stroudsburg University of Pennsylvania (ESU), Scanton, Pennsylvania, US

The purpose of developing the dual-degree MD/Master of Public Health program (MD/MPH) and the MD/Public Health Certificate (MD/PHC) program between The Commonwealth Medical College and East Stroudsburg University is to enrich the education of future primary care physicians, teachers, and researchers by developing and integrating a public health curriculum within traditional medical education. The partnership between TCMC, a new community-health and public-health focused allopathic (MD) medical school in rural northeastern Pennsylvania (NEPA) and ESU's public health programs will ultimately improve health outcomes and reduce health disparities in the regions our students serve. CEPH is an independent agency recognized by the US Department of Education to accredit public health programs. Educational training in public health is essential to better address the health inequities endemic experienced in our geographic region, which includes an aging population, a high rate of childhood poverty, and disproportionately high rates of cancer, cardiovascular disease

* Correspondence: Mark V White, MD, MPH, Department of Family, Community, and Rural Health, Associate Professor of Epidemiology, The Commonwealth Medical College, 525 Pine Street, Scranton, PA 18509, United States. E-mail: mwhite@tcmedc.org.

and mental illness. Residents of NEPA are experiencing access to care issues, especially related to primary care, mental health, and dental care.

Introduction

Practitioners, educators, and researchers working in the fields of public health and primary care strive for the common goal of improved health of individuals and their communities. Despite this mutual aim, the efforts of primary care physicians and public health practitioners are often disconnected from one another, to the detriment of their patients and communities. In a healthcare environment characterized by marked policy change, limited resources, and increasing need, the fields of primary care and public health will require more support from one another. A symbiotic relationship between these fields that involves inter-professional collaborations, community engagement, and collaborative evidence-based research endeavors will be essential to the achievement of the mutual goals of enhanced primary care and improved community health.

Medical schools provide natural opportunities to integrate public health training and primary care. To this end, The Commonwealth Medical College (TCMC) and East Stroudsburg University of Pennsylvania (ESU), both located in Northeastern Pennsylvania (NEPA), have collaborated to develop a curriculum that infuses public health training, community engagement, and inter-professional collaboration into traditional medical education. This collaboration has led to the development of two new programs: a Public Health Certificate (PHC) or a Master of Public Health (MPH) degree, available to TCMC medical students. These programs will prepare participants to make significant contributions to the healthcare environment in which they eventually practice, including increased access to quality health care and improved population health.

Current state of health care in the region

There is a shortage of primary care physicians in Pennsylvania, particularly in the northeast region. Presently, PA retains only 22% of its physician trainees and of these only: 16% practice primary care; 7% practice rural care; 4% practice rural primary care; and 0.5% practice rural underserved care.

Additionally, PA currently ranks 37th in the US in physicians per 10,000 elderly persons. The average age of physicians in Pennsylvania is 48.7, with those under 35 years of age consisting of only 8% of the physician workforce. Further, 21% of physicians currently practicing state that they will stop practicing within five years (1).

TCMC serves 16 counties, whose population ranges from 6,124 (Sullivan) to 311,983 (Luzerne). Only Lackawanna and Luzerne have significant "urban" centers- Scranton, population 72,233, and Wilkes-Barre, population 40,932; yet both counties have many rural communities. Williamsport, population 29,456, is the county seat for Pennsylvania's largest county, Lycoming County, which is rural.

The majority of 16 counties in TCMC's coverage region include federally designated shortage areas for primary care, dental, and/or mental health professionals. The residents of

TCMC's region are disproportionately affected by mental health challenges and a lack of access, and experience high rates of obesity, heart disease, and other chronic diseases (2).

A Regional Health Needs Assessment conducted in 2009 by the Department of Family, Community and Rural Health (DFCRH) showed that mental health, transportation problems, lack of health insurance, lack of providers, lack of preventive care, drug and alcohol abuse, cultural and knowledge barriers to care and oral health care were areas of need. Interagency collaboration, the State Health Improvement Plan (SHIP) partnerships, volunteers, schools and churches as pillars of community were noted as strengths (3).

In 23 focus groups representative of 195 community agencies, participants reported mental health as a predominant concern in each county, and large gaps in mental health services: a lack of psychiatrists, scarce children's mental health services, long waiting lists and waits for appointments, lack of services for patients with concomitant substance abuse, and an enormous burden on primary care physicians and social service agencies trying to fill the gap. Isolation and depression, leading to poor physical health were identified as a major problem among seniors in the region. Lackawanna, Luzerne, and Schuylkill counties have very high youth suicide rate (3). The findings have been published (3,4) and will continue to be used to guide development of the research, educational and clinical agendas of TCMC.

Public health education initiatives, such as this inter-professional dual degree program, encourage students to invest their time, energy, and efforts to approach patient care with a public health perspective. The theoretical framework for the programs is based on accountability to the public good, specifically in the NEPA region. The principles and practice of Community Based Participatory Research (CBPR), the World Health Organization's International Classification of Function, Disability, and Health (ICF) and social ecology models inform the curriculum and assessment strategies. Graduates of these programs will be equipped for positions in health departments, federally qualified health centers, and other organizations that require expertise in prevention strategies and healthcare policy.

Goals and objectives

The main objective of the PHC and MPH programs is to provide training in environmental health, infectious disease control, disease prevention, health promotion, epidemiology, and injury control. TCMC is committed to the integration of community and public health in medical education, and these programs expand upon the standard curriculum, integrating population health skills, experiences, and core public health competencies that guide clinical practice and lead to improved access to quality care. Through ESU's MPH program, TCMC offers medical students a unique opportunity to receive a well-rounded curriculum in public health. The partnership between these two institutions will ultimately contribute to improving health outcomes and reduce health disparities in the regions the graduates ultimately serve.

Our project

The Commonwealth Medical College (TCMC) is located in northeast and north central Pennsylvania and offers a community-based model of medical education with three regional campuses - North (Scranton), South (Wilkes-Barre), and West (Williamsport). The College was awarded degree granting authority by the Commonwealth of Pennsylvania in 2008, received preliminary LCME (Liaison Committee on Medical Education) accreditation in 2008; provisional accreditation in 2012, and accepted its first class of medical and master's students in 2009.

The four year MD Program features team and case-based learning, inter-professional education, early exposure to clinical care settings, medical simulation, standardized patients, and community health and research projects. TCMC is among the first United States medical schools to adopt the Longitudinal Integrated Clerkship (LIC) model as the standard clinical experience for the entire medical school class in the third year. As the core of the LIC, TCMC incorporates longitudinal ambulatory clerkships within each of the six core disciplines: medicine, surgery, pediatrics, psychiatry, obstetrics and gynecology, and family medicine. Students in these clerkships follow panels of patients longitudinally with their faculty. Interspersed with these longitudinal ambulatory half-days are group and case-based learning sessions and tutorials, inpatient rounds, emergency room experiences and self-directed learning.

The College attracts students from across the nation who are interested in studying evidence- and community-based medicine and who have a strong desire to serve their community. The students have early clinical experiences and are engaged with clinical mentors right from the start of their medical education. Each of the three campuses offers exposure to urban and rural settings and diverse clinical experiences. Medical students receive regional campus assignments following matriculation and are paired with community physicians who serve as continuity mentors throughout their education.

The Department of Family, Community, and Rural Health (DFCRH) played a major role in curriculum development for the medical school and faculty members conduct public health, epidemiologic and clinical research. Relationships with various community agencies became crucial when incorporating Community Health Research Projects (CHRPs) in the first year and the Family Centered Experience across the four years of the standard medical education curriculum. Advantages of being a newer institution include the opportunities for flexibility and innovation for faculty and students. There was a tremendous amount of institutional support for public health training at TCMC, a key factor in establishing these programs (5).

East Stroudsburg University of Pennsylvania

ESU is one of 14 state-supported institutions in the Pennsylvania State System of Higher Education (PASSHE), and is accredited by the Middle States Association of Colleges and Schools. The institution's MPH program, housed within ESU's Department of Health Studies, was approved by PASSHE in 1988 and has been continuously accredited by the Council on Education in Public Health (CEPH) since 1990. The MPH program at ESU consists of 45 credits aimed at preparing students in the core public health competencies (Epidemiology, Health Administration, Environmental Health, Social and Behavioral Sciences, and Biostatistics).

Requirements include a 300 hour internship requirement, a publishable paper and a comprehensive oral exam. An 18-credit Certificate of Public Health primarily for professionals working in the health and social services sectors is also available. This curriculum emphasizes population-based approaches, strengthening capacity for community-based prevention in order to promote healthy behaviors, and using environmental change strategies to enhance health and impact policy.

ESU public health programs aim to prepare the public health workforce to partner with communities while promoting collaboration and empowerment. The MPH and the public health certificate programs at ESU include training in cultural competency, addressing health disparities, use of technology in health care, and research methodology. Application of these skills to real-world scenarios during the required internship experience is an essential component of both programs.

Funding

Initial discussions and planning meetings involved key stakeholders from both institutions. A grant application was submitted to the Health Resources and Services Administration (HRSA) and TCMC were awarded funding in the amount of $1.5 million (T85HP24464) over a five-year period, with ESU and the NEPA Area Health Education Center (AHEC) as subcontractors. This grant provides partial tuition for students and also supports faculty time spent mentoring, preparing, advising, researching, and teaching public health students.

Program description

The ESU Master of Public Health program prepares students to enter the field of public health as researchers and practitioners working in the prevention of disease and improvement of the quality of life in communities. Through a well-integrated program of study, students receive instruction in the core public health disciplines of Biostatistics, Environmental Health, Epidemiology, Health Policy & Administration, and Social and Behavioral Sciences.

Students have opportunities to explore the intersection of the social behavioral sciences, information technology, human biology, and policy development. They have practical experiences in policy development, practice-based research, and program implementation. These internships are required to complete both the certificate and master's programs.

The challenge was to combine curricula from two separate institutions into one dual degree program. Please refer to Table 1 for a curriculum layout for all medical students pursuing either a MPH or PHC. It details the five year plan to infuse public health classes into the standard TCMC curriculum.

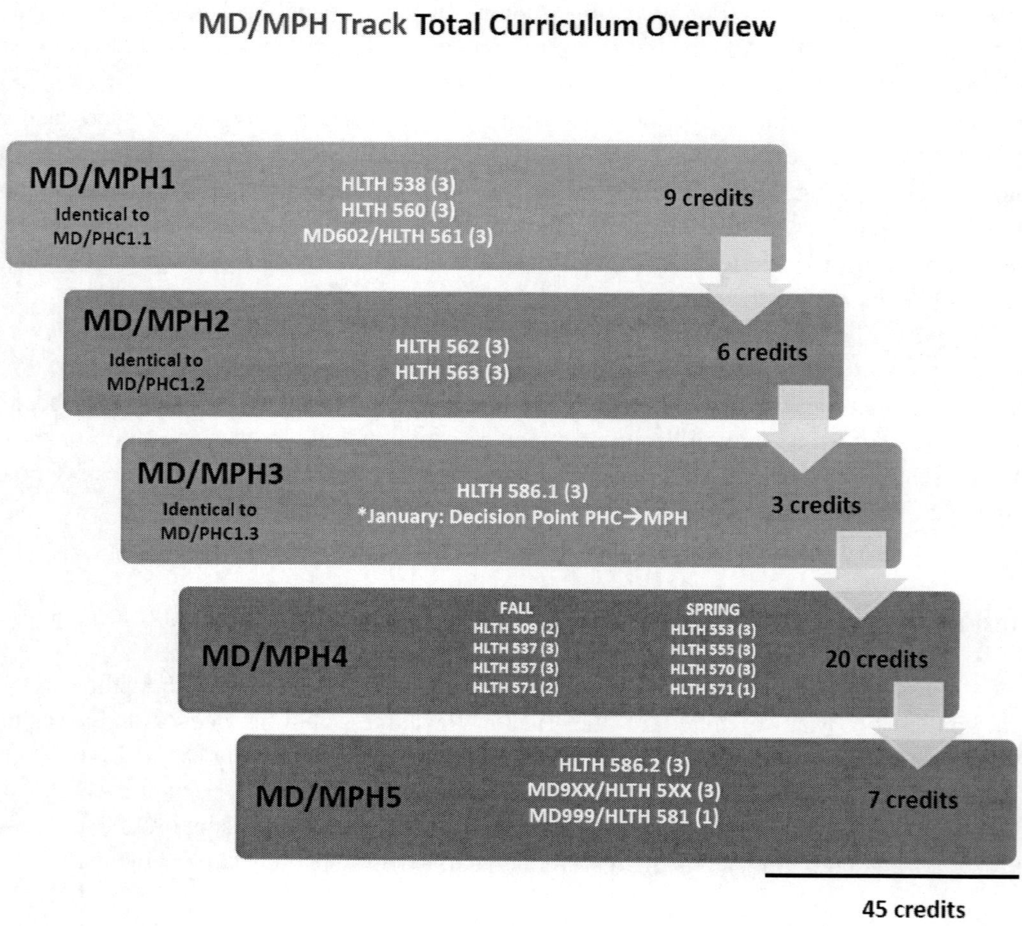

Figure 1. Curriculum Overview.

Both programs require internship experiences in a public health field to complete their certificate or degree requirements. TCMC and ESU have relationships with community leaders and healthcare providers dedicated to furthering public health in the communities which serve as internship sites for students.

How program addresses health needs

The establishment of TCMC, with its core mission of primary care training, has facilitated collaboration among research and health entities in NEPA to create an infrastructure that can effectively address the health disparities in the region. The collaboration with ESU allows TCMC to further integrate public health into primary care training. Previous collaborations with county-level State Health Improvement Plan Partners (SHIPs) and with community research areas have resulted in a "workforce" that is ready to address public health issues on a more systemic level.

For example, TCMC faculty and students have supported a community task force in Schuylkill County with their efforts at establishing a community health center (CHC). They have also assisted in creating the non-profit corporation that can evolve into a CHC, conducted surveys and are currently exploring the establishment of a medical reserve corps that can address public health needs in the county. It is anticipated that medical students in the public health training programs will be placed in meaningful internships in Schuylkill County to support these efforts. Other examples of community agencies that TCMC partners with include the Northeast Pennsylvania Cancer Research Institute, Wayne Memorial Hospital and the Children's Advocacy Center. These and numerous other partnerships will provide potential sites for student internships.

Strengthening existing community partnerships

A variety of community-based research, quality improvement, and summer research projects are essential components of TCMC's strategy to emphasize the value of community engagement and community partnerships within an allopathic medical curriculum. First-year medical students at TCMC are required to complete a Community Health Research Project (CHRP) as a component of the "Physician and Society" course, where many core principles of public health are introduced. These projects involve a group of students working in collaboration with both an internal TCMC mentor and an external community agency or organization to contribute to improved health in the region by applying the concepts, strategies, and tools acquired in their studies (4).

Over the past five years, CHRPs have been conducted with a cadre of varied community agencies throughout NEPA, including the Northeast Regional Cancer Institute, the Lupus Foundation, the Lackawanna County Library System, Children's Advocacy Center, Volunteers in Medicine, the Care and Concern Clinic, and many more. The topics and scope of these projects change year to year depending upon the community partner agency and the type of research planned. Each student group prepares and presents an academic poster documenting the rationale, research design, data analysis, and discussion of their project during an annual Research Symposium event, to which all of the current and past partnering community agencies are invited. Multi-year CHRPs involving several stages/types of research on the same broad topic with the same community agencies are currently planned to further strengthen these existing community partnerships in an effort to maximize the impact on and benefit to the students and community partners involved.

Community engagement and inter-professional collaboration are again emphasized in the second year of TCMC's MD curriculum, when students are required to complete a Quality Improvement Community Collaborative (QuICC) project as a component of the "Art and Practice of Medicine" course. Working in groups, second-year medical students partner with a community-based team of health care professionals to measurably improve some aspect of patient care in a clinical setting. QuICC projects utilize the "Plan-Do-Study-Act" quality improvement cycle, and have focused on topics such as geriatric care, hand washing and vaccination rates, and guideline compliance for Pap smears, Constant Positive Airway Pressure (CPAP) use, and blood pressure monitoring. The settings for these projects range from small rural practices to busy hospital sites.

Often, the same community agencies and institutions that are collaborators for CHRPs are able to mentor QuICC projects as well; this internal consistency will augment alliances with community partners. As with the first-year CHRPs, student groups prepare and present academic posters at TCMC's annual Research Symposium event. In addition to presentation to the TCMC community, many students involved in CHRP and QuICC projects have gone on to present their posters at national academic or professional conferences such as TCMC Annual Research Symposium, Pennsylvania Academy of Family Physicians (PAFP) conference, and American College of Physician's (ACP) annual meeting.

Findings

There are currently four TCMC medical students enrolled in the MD/public health program. They are the participants of the pilot program and have completed the first two semesters of the curriculum.

Recruitment

Recruitment is a crucial part of the success of any academic program. Recruitment strategies included partnering with student affairs and encouraging the enrolled students to serve as ambassadors for the programs. In the first year, recruitment was somewhat challenging as can be expected for any new program. The TCMC MD/MPH program coordinator was hired, whose responsibilities included student recruitment, assisting prospective students with the application process, and writing reports on all grant-related activities. In the future, prospective students applying to TCMC will receive information about the public health training programs, with the expectation that such opportunities will positively influence recruitment into the MD program. TCMC and ESU are exploring creative methods of marketing the program to current and prospective students.

The public health programs have been highlighted during admissions interviews, orientation and at other events, such as the TCMC revisit day, greatly increasing their exposure. Coordination of efforts between TCMC's Offices of Student Affairs, Academic Affairs, Marketing and Public Relations, and Curriculum has created a multi-tiered recruitment strategy with promising results.

Members of the newly-created Public Health Student Association will take an active role as recruitment ambassadors for the program, and create a mentorship program for those students newer to public health. Current MD/Public Health program students will also present a panel at a monthly Lunch and Learn seminar which is open to all students, faculty, and staff. Students will be encouraged to stay committed to the curriculum, create an internal support system and serve as ambassadors for public health within the institution.

Discussion

Lack of lead time in recruitment during the first grant year limited the number of students enrolled in the program. When the HRSA grant was awarded, the team worked as quickly as possible to launch classes in July of 2013. The brief amount of time between the date of the grant award and the beginning of ESU coursework presented a barrier to acclimating students to the public health programs. All accepted students planned a visit to TCMC in the spring before their first year of medical school. The coordinators and faculty at that point reached out to the pre-matriculating students about the benefits of the programs. Due to limited exposure to the pre-matriculating students, enrollment for the pilot year of the programs was lower than anticipated.

A second challenge to recruitment is the time commitment needed for students pursuing an MD/MPH dual degree. Students must plan on a fifth year of study and are required to make significant personal, professional and financial commitments to the program early on in their medical training. Prospective students had concerns about graduating with their classmates and workload manageability during their first year of medical school. Two of the first group of enrollees dropped out shortly after enrolling.

Evaluation plans

The evaluation plan includes assessment of students' attainment of specific competencies in public health. Both quantitative and qualitative methodologies will be employed. TCMC's Department of Curriculum Development and Assessment will oversee program evaluation.

Student attitudes and perceptions will be assessed using data derived from questionnaires and focus groups; fund of knowledge from National Board of Medical Examiners (NBME) Subject Exams and NBME Comprehensive Clinical Science Self Assessments (CCSSA). The Jefferson Scale of Physician Empathy (JSPE) will be completed at the beginning and the end of the academic year, which will allow 'empathy erosion' to be measured and compared over time. Students' career interests will be surveyed yearly to track changes over time using an internally administered survey, beginning with pre-matriculation to the MD Curriculum. Students' attitudes to primary care will also be assessed prior to the beginning of the LIC and after completion of the LIC. In addition, TCMC will survey graduates at 1 and every 5 years after completion of their medical education regarding career choice, primary care practice, and practice in HPSAs, MUAs or other underserved communities/populations as well as level of community engagement/public health activities. Residency directors will be surveyed during TCMC graduate's internship year to assess overall competence and qualities such as patient and community centeredness, team skills, and cultural competence.

Dissemination plans

It is anticipated that information about these collaborative programs will be disseminated at various national and international conferences, as well as through additional peer-reviewed publications.

Future plans

Additional funding will be sought to ensure sustainability of the program beyond the five year funding period. It is anticipated that institutional funds from both partners will continue to be available to support the program. Potential modifications to the program include making more courses available online to facilitate scheduling and reduce costs. (Currently, a modest number of courses are offered online). Additional partnerships with community agencies will be sought out in order to provide more practical opportunities for students while fulfilling the missions of both institutions.

Table 1. Acronyms Used

TCMC	The Commonwealth Medical College
ESU	East Stroudsburg University
MPH	Master's of Public Health
PHC	Public Health Certificate
LIC	Longitudinal Integrated Curriculum
CPAP	Constant Positive Airway Pressure
NBME	National Board of Medical Examiners
CHRP	Community Health Research Project
QuICC	Quality Improvement Community Collaborative Project
NEPA	Northeastern Pennsylvania
CCSSA	Comprehensive Clinical Science Self Assessments
JSPE	Jefferson Scale of Physician Empathy
DFCRH	Department of Family, Community and Rural Health
SHIP	State Health Improvement Plan
CEPH	Council on Education for Public Health
DFCRH	Department of Family, Community and Rural Health
HPSAs	Health Professional Shortage Areas
MUAs	Medically Underserved Areas
HRSA	Health Resources and Services Association
ICF	International Classification of Function, Disability, and Health
PASSHE	Pennsylvania State System of Higher Education
AHEC	Area Health Education Center
PAFP	Pennsylvania Academy of Family Physicians
LCME	Liaison Committee on Medical Education
ACP	American College of Physicians

Acknowledgments

Funding for this project was made possible in part by T85HP24464 from the Health Resources and Services Administration. The views expressed do not necessarily reflect the official policies of the Department of Health and Human Services nor does mention of trade names, commercial practices, or organizations imply endorsement by the US Government.

References

[1] Quraishi SA, Orkin FK, Weitekamp MR, Khalid AN, Sassani JW. The health policy and legislative awareness initiative at the Pennsylvania State University college of medicine: theory meets practice. Acad Med 2005;80(5):443-7.

[2] Pennsylvania Department of Health. Pennsylvania: EpiQMS. Regional Health Statistics. Accessed 2012 April 14. URL: http://www.portal.state.pa.us/portal/server.pt?open=514&objID= 596553& mode=2

[3] Garrettson M, Walline V, Heisler J, Townsend J. New medical school engages rural communities to conduct regional health assessment. Fam Med 2010;42(10):693-701.

[4] Simoyan OM, Townsend JM, Tarafder MR, DeJoseph D, Stark RJ, White MV. Public and medical education: a natural alliance for a new regional medical school. Am J Prev Med 2011;41(4S3): S220-7.

[5] Simoyan OM, Townsend JM. Improving the health of northeastern Pennsylvania through medical education and community engagement. Public Voices 2012;12(2):38-48.

In: Public Health
Editors: Rosemary M. Caron and Joav Merrick

ISBN: 978-1-63321-569-6

Chapter 4

Building inter-professional cultural competence

Joy Doll*[*], *Ann Ryan Haddad, Ann Laughlin, Martha Todd, Katie Packard, Jennifer Yee, Barbara Harris and Kimberly Begley
Department of Occupational Therapy, Department of Pharmacy Practice, College of Nursing, Department of Exercise Science, Department of Social Work, Creighton University, Omaha, Nebraska, US

Inter-professional education (IPE) necessitates that both educators and students need to engage in a process that requires learning and reflecting upon professional identity, both their own and those of the other professionals on the healthcare team. Despite thinking team skills are inherent, it has become apparent that health professions students need to be taught the skills of how to communicate and negotiate as part of a team to provide collaborative care. These skills demand that health care providers need to not only learn discipline-specific clinical reasoning but team-based clinical reasoning as well. The Inter-professional Education Collaborative Expert Panel has clearly identified team-based skills as a core skill to health care practice. Teamwork and team-based skills become even more critical in health care delivery for vulnerable patients and populations. Vulnerable patients present with complex health issues that benefit from a team-based approach to care. This chapter will describe the development and implementation of a pilot IPE course preparing students for health care with vulnerable patients. The authors discuss the importance of developing inter-professional cultural competence for the faculty team of educators in order to execute such complex IPE. Reflections on the challenges to developing and implementing such an innovative IPE experience will be discussed.

[*] Corresponding author: Joy Doll, OTD, OTR/L, Vice Chair, Director of Post Professional OTD Program, Associate Professor, Department of Occupational Therapy, School of Pharmacy and Health Professions, Creighton University, 2500 California Plaza, Omaha, Nebraska, United States. E-mail: joydoll@creighton.edu.

Introduction

Scholars, educators and health care organizations all agree: inter-professional education (IPE) and collaborative health care practice are essential to provide quality, holistic care for patients across health care settings (1). Health care providers today are faced with challenges including complex diagnoses and limited resources along with providing care in a diverse team environment to maximize care. The importance of team care becomes more evident when working with patients who are vulnerable. Collaborative care and team-based practice are now being recognized as skills that need to be taught and enhanced (1). Health care team interactions that are negative or ineffective can profoundly impact patient outcomes and the overall success of a health care organization (2). Team development, both for the individual health care practitioner and the health care team, is also critical to the success of collaborative care (2). Inter-professional education (IPE) has emerged as a pedagogical approach to train health care students to be prepared for health care practice. Within the context of IPE, a variety of pedagogies have been shown to teach collaborative, team skills. The overall intent of IPE is to move students beyond thinking within one's own health care discipline and to expand clinical reasoning to a team-based approach (3).

Accreditation bodies have now included inter-professional practice as a core skill for many health care professions (4,5). Students from across the health sciences will now be learning skills including collaborative ethical decision making, how to engage in successful team interactions, appropriate team communication and team problem solving (1). Pecukonis, Doyle, and Bliss (6) propose that the best way to prepare students to build the skills necessary for collaborative care in practice is to develop inter-professional cultural competence. Despite an effort in IPE to build team-based care skills, health care education is largely "profession-centric" which leads to the development of ethnocentrism held by professionals creating barriers to collaborative health care practice (6).

According to Pecukonis et al. (6), even the social construction of the term "professionalism" does not promote collaboration but instead leads to competition among health care providers. Due to the social construct of being part of a profession, collaborative care faces challenges and requires health professions educators to alter their thinking to develop and implement appropriate IPE. In order to break down existing social constructs to promote increased collaborative care, Pecukonis et al. proposed that educators follow the concept of IDEA: Interaction, Data, Expertise and Attention (6). The authors of this manuscript will use the mnemonic of IDEA to describe the development of an IPE course focused on preparing students, both as individuals and as part of a team, to provide care to vulnerable populations and/or individuals. The premise of IDEA provides a foundation for building inter-professional cultural competence not just among students but professionals and educators as well. Experts in inter-professional education have long argued the importance of faculty development for successful IPE (7). Any team of educators implementing IPE need to develop their own inter-professional cultural competence in order to be effective in designing and implementing successful IPE for students. This manuscript will describe the journey of a team of educators in developing inter-professional cultural competence while facing the challenges of developing an IPE course focused on vulnerable populations.

Intersecting inter-professional education and vulnerability

Simulation centers, service-learning, case analysis, and patient safety have all been exemplars in teaching health professions students the skills necessary to engage in collaborative health care practice (3,4,10). However, as identified by Dow et al. (9), one area of inter-professional education still in need of development is the preparation of the inter-professional team for working with vulnerable and/or underserved populations. According to Dow et al. (9) "a student planning to practice in a resource-poor, primary care setting needs specific skills in teamwork, leadership, and followership that bolster collaboration by allowing all health care professionals to practice at the top of their licensed abilities" (9). In fact, these leaders in IPE identify the skills for working as part of an inter-professional team with a vulnerable population as one of the existing challenges facing current inter-professional education (9). But a question remains: how do we prepare health professions students to graduate prepared with the skills to collaborate in a team specifically focused on the needs of a vulnerable and/or underserved population? Dow, et al., suggest that educational institutions need to partner with health care organizations where both entities work together "to devise curriculum and measure outcomes" (9). Based on this identified gap in IPE, educators are called to develop educational opportunities to prepare students to practice in underserved areas.

Vulnerability can be described in a multitude of ways and is confounded in health care by factors such as chronic disease, poverty, low health literacy rates, uninsured and underinsured health care insurance coverage, and health disparities. These issues are further exacerbated by limited English proficiency, cultural beliefs and underrepresentation of minorities in health care provision (10,11). Multiple factors related to vulnerability can result in increasing the complexity of health care decision making for the individual health professional and the health care team. Eamon (12) defined a vulnerable population as "a group possessing a disproportionate amount of societal resources and influence". Vulnerable populations are "at risk of discrimination, oppression, possessing few social and economic resources and exclusion from decision-making processes" (12). Across the literature, there are examples of IPE experiences have taken place with ethnic minorities and rural populations where community leaders and educators have felt that inter-professional practice is necessary to address the needs of vulnerable populations. These experiences often focus on identified "underserved populations," who experience vulnerability due to health disparities and geographic isolation (13).

Student-run clinics in underserved communities have been one avenue for exposing students to IPE with vulnerable populations (14). Students report enjoying these experiences as a way to collaborate and meet community needs (15). Educational experiences with underserved populations also allow students the opportunity to learn the importance of overlapping roles and how to collaborate with limited resources to meet patient needs (16). However, to develop and sustain these inter-professional experiences for students, academicians have to be committed to collaborative work, crossing professional boundaries and possess a willingness to grow as a team (17). It bears stating that any team of educators implementing IPE need to experience team development and effective collaboration in order to effectively educate teams of health professions students (18). In other words the team of faculty developing and implementing IPE needs to develop inter-professional cultural competence among its member and the team as a whole. To achieve IPE, each faculty member must confront and identify how to distribute "power within the work environment, how training should proceed within the clinical setting, the level, and nature of inter-profession communication, resolution of conflicts and management of relationships between team members and constituents" (6).

When developing a team, educators and students alike are called to explore their own vulnerabilities in order to identify and develop inter-professional cultural competence. Although this vulnerability is different than the vulnerabilities of the underserved, the exposure to these feelings can be a catalyst to the openness needed by both the educators and the students to effectively work as a team with vulnerable patients. Furthermore, the members of a health care team should experience their own vulnerability in order to reflect and grow into a strong collaborative team. All of these elements are critical in order for an individual and a team to develop inter-professional cultural competence (18).

Interaction: Formulating the course design

According to Pecukonis et al. interaction "is the process during which the student has the opportunity to work and learn directly with individuals from other health disciplines" (6). The same principle is as true for health sciences educators, as it is for students. The educators involved in developing the inter-professional course exemplar discussed here had a longstanding relationship with one another. Prior to the course development and implementation, these educators had collaborated on the execution of an inter-professional clinic for the underserved in a low socioeconomic area lacking in health care services. The clinic resulted from a group of passionate and committed faculty who were compelled to interact to make the clinic a successful reality. Through these interactions surrounding the clinic, faculty engaged in collaborative communication, role negotiation, knowledgeable transition about professions on the team, and developed a sense of advocacy for all the various professions involved. These activities are critical in the process of developing inter-professional cultural competence (6).

To maintain the demands of the clinic, faculty and student volunteers took responsibility for the day-to-day management of the clinic. From the faculty experience with the students, the educators identified a need to formalize the education occurring at the community partner site to structure learning experiences and prepare students for the realities of the needs and desires of vulnerable clients. Faculty observations and conversations revealed a significant lack of knowledge demonstrated by students regarding how to address the needs of the vulnerable population being served at the clinic. Furthermore, the students were observed to have a lack of clear awareness of how to act and interact as part of a health care team. From these observations and discussions, the idea of an inter-professional course focused on developing the skills necessary to provide collaborative care for vulnerable populations emerged. It is significant to point out that the inter-professional team of faculty had to collaborate and engage in open dialogue in order to clearly identify the educational needs of the students. The interactions from the clinic established clear team interactions and allowed the team to identify the need to grow inter-professional education experiences for the students.

Table 1. IDEA constructs for inter-professional cultural competence

Construct	Description
Interaction	Educators will: • Expose to students and professionals from different health professions to develop knowledge about professional practices across professions • Have students learning in collaboration with other professions forcing students to challenge professional beliefs and move towards inter-professional cultural competence
Data	Educators will: • Facilitate students to ask and seek information about other health care professions to understand their profession's role in accordance with the roles of other professions on the health care team • Help students explore stereotypes and biases they hold about professions' roles including their own • Provide activities that allow students to develop relationships with students from other professions to see them not just as professionals, but a person
Expertise	Educators will: • Encourage the development of skills in collaborative communication and reflective practices in order to develop an increased awareness of others in order to promote collaborative care
Attention	Educators will: • Provide opportunities for students to reflect both personally and as a team on their own beliefs about professions' roles and team-based care

Data: Course design and implementation

In the IDEA mnemonic, Data focuses on "obtaining accurate information from health professions" (6). In order to cultivate the IPE course, the faculty began to meet and collaborate on the course design which included the development of the course syllabus and exploration into the administrative infrastructure for the approval of such a course. The course was designed by the team of faculty involved in the clinic from the professions of exercise science, occupational therapy, nursing, pharmacy and social work. Each faculty member then recruited students from these professions to engage in the course. As part of the process, faculty developed a strong understanding of the roles of other team members to formulate how the course would be presented. To role model collaborative care to students, the educators, themselves, had to learn about one another and negotiate their own collaborative process.

The team of faculty was also required to navigate the institutional infrastructure required to implement an IPE course which necessitated the team members to acquire new knowledge. For the course to be approved and categorized as IPE, a copy of the syllabus had to be reviewed and accepted by the curriculum committees of each profession involved at the institution. The team of faculty designing the course was responsible for contacting the appropriate representatives and garnering support to receive approval from all the curriculum committees. In one discipline, the curriculum committee did not approve the course so students from this discipline had to be excluded from the enrollment. Furthermore, IPE courses are a workload add-on at the institution and not currently recognized in a faculty's current teaching duties. This situation forced the team members to negotiate with administrators and those on the team to identify a time to hold the course sessions that worked for all involved, both students and instructors. Due to workload issues, the team decided to limit the enrollment of students to 8 health professions students in order to pilot the course and ensure its successful implementation. Team members also took responsibility for teaching certain modules in an effort to manage faculty workload. In overcoming logistical challenges, the team members had to understand all team members' roles advocating for one another to ensure the course could take place. Understanding the roles of each member on the team was critical to ensure successful collaboration and a positive course experience for all involved.

Another component of data is "developing both insight and understanding about the person one is working with" (6). The successful design and implementation of this course was generated out of the passion of a group of faculty who care for one another and those who are vulnerable, not only as professionals and patients, but as people. These underpinnings of teamwork can be misconstrued as too qualitative and are often undervalued (19). However, the authors of this manuscript feel that the elements of compassion and empathy are sorely underscored in many IPE endeavors (20). This compassion among team members led to the consideration of many small, yet important, elements in the course design like the need to implement the course off campus. The rationale for holding the course in the community was to ensure the students gained a "real world" experience outside the sheltered context of the university.

Upon designing the course, faculty had to obtain administrative approval from the university to offer a full course off campus and also coordinate with the community site to choose a time that worked for the partner, the students' and the educators' schedules. In order to allow collaboration and address schedule conflicts, the course was designed as a hybrid learning experience requiring some learning in the community and some in an online environment. The instructors found both interactions to be rich in nature demonstrating the importance of care for team members in all contexts. Although often undervalued, caring for one another allowed the team, both of faculty and students, to interact effectively and maintain momentum despite some arduous barriers. This led to Expertise, the next component in cultivating inter-professional cultural competence.

Expertise and attention: Build competence to implement successful IPE

Expertise entails "the ability to communicate clearly, and effectively with other disciplines concerning the values and processes of patient care" (6). In order to develop and implement the course, the educators had to be efficient collaborators which included communicating with team members and beyond. In addition to Expertise, the team had to engage in extensive critical reflection, both individually and as a team, which addresses the aspect of Attention of the IDEA mnemonic. Attention "involves the in-depth exploration of one's personal, professional and cultural background" along with recognizing and trying to understand the biases and assumptions carried by others on the team (6).

Negotiating workload concerns was an issue that required significant communication among the faculty team members in planning the course. Discussing team members' perceptions and assumptions was an important part of the process to help the team collaborate. These negotiations required the team to engage in both Expertise and Attention to develop team competence. During the class sessions, all the instructors involved in the course made a concerted effort to be on site to role model inter-professionalism to the student inter-professional teams. Once students were given their case and charged with meeting in their teams to develop care plans, the instructors were available for both discipline-specific and inter-professional interactions as consultants. This infrastructure was necessary in order to role model and help the students build skills in communication for the progress of their own inter-professional cultural competence.

It is important to note that ventures, such as the design and implementation of an IPE course of this nature, require significant faculty time commitment and passion. Furthermore, the development and maintenance of the team aligns with the concept of Expertise which "requires compromise, embracing the others perspectives" (6). To design the course framework, the team of faculty met many times to discuss the course lessons. There were zealous discussions about course content and how it should be delivered. Critical to the success of this collaborative design was the prior establishment of a strong team of inter-professional faculty where members felt free to voice their thoughts and opinions. The process of dialogue and compromise led to the development of a course that met the requirements of multiple health professions and the passions of the team of faculty involved in the course. The ultimate goal of implementing IPE to train future health professions for intervening with vulnerable populations was realized due to the faculty team's concerted effort to foster and build inter-professional cultural competence.

IDEA: Student formation of inter-professional cultural competence

Eight students were selected to be enrolled in the pilot IPE course focused on vulnerable populations. Upon completion, the course was entitled "Developing Care for a Vulnerable Population: An Inter-professional Collaborative Approach for Health Promotion." Health professions students from the disciplines of nursing (n=2), occupational therapy (n=2), pharmacy (n=2), social work (n=1) and exercise science (n=1) were recruited by faculty investigators in the semester prior to starting the course. In some professions, there was a large interest in the course and the faculty had to gather to choose the students for the course. When this was the case, the instructors selected students whom they felt would be committed to the course and held a strong desire to serve with vulnerable populations as part of their future professional practice.

The course met for eight weeks focused on acclimating students to their discipline. The students were divided into two 4-member teams mixing up the disciplines. Prior to collaborating with clients, students also engaged in course activities learning about the role of their discipline with a vulnerable population, the role of the other disciplines on the team, exploring the context of vulnerability, evaluating case scenarios, and promoting inter-professional dialogue and interactions between both students and faculty. The students engaged in learning activities, discussed team skills, and developed a collaborative agreement for how the team would interact to serve the vulnerable client.

In partnership with the community, two community members who had been reoccurring users of the clinic and currently experiencing complex health issues were invited to participate as the clients for the course. The community members were each invited to a live classroom session at the community partner site to share their experience with the health care system and their health concerns with both teams. The teams were then each assigned one of the community members who were considered part of their team. Students, with faculty supervision, conducted further assessment of the community member with their consent and developed a collaborative care plan for the client. Students were encouraged to reflect both individually and as a team. In group reflection discussions, students reported surprise at the complexities of the issues, both health and social, experienced by the community members who volunteered to work with the students.

In order to gauge the impact of the course and focus on the growth in inter-professional cultural competence, the faculty spent time reflecting on this pilot both during and after the course, which led to course modification and the formation of this manuscript. Quantitative data was also collected from the student participants to assess the impact of the course on their learning. This data was important to evaluate the effect on the learning of the group of inter-professional health professions students enrolled in the course. It was hypothesized that after completing the course, student perceptions about working as part of a team would improve. The study was reviewed and approved by the University Social/Behavioral Institutional Review Board.

At the beginning and end of the course, students completed the Team Skills Scale (21). Questions for the Team Skills Scale were drawn from the John A Hartford Foundation, Geriatric Interdisciplinary Team Training Program (GITT) kit (22). The scale measures perception of capabilities for effective team interactions and consists of 17 questions at 5 points each, for a maximum score of 85 points. The scale was originally designed to measure three key areas: interpersonal skills, profession-specific skills, and geriatric care skills. Questions are answered on a Likert scale measuring 1 = poor, 2 = fair, 3 = good,4 = very good, and 5 = excellent.

Data from the pre- and post- student surveys were analyzed using Microsoft Excel using paired student's t tests. A *p*-value less than .05 was considered statistically significant. There was a non-significant increase in the mean Team Skills Scale score (70.0 ± 11.1 pre versus 75.9 ± 13.0 post, $p=0.09$) (Table 2).

Though the data show trends in perceived improvement of skills needed to work as part of an inter-professional team, statistical significance may not have been achieved due to small sample size (n=8). Likewise, it has been shown that students new to inter-professional experiences often overestimate their baseline team skills, which may explain why several of the students showed a decrease in their overall score post intervention (23). These data show that a semester long inter-professional course in caring for vulnerable populations may improve students' perceptions of their abilities to work as part of an inter-professional team. It may begin the journey for health professions students in gaining inter-professional cultural competence. As the course is replicated in subsequent semesters, the sample size will increase to determine if this is a significant finding. Despite the lack of significance, the faculty involved in the course feel that the lessons learned about implementing such an IPE experience cannot be undervalued. The authors feel that the journey to inter-professional cultural competence is a story worth telling to demonstrate the complexities and intricacies of IPE for vulnerable populations.

Table 2. Team Skills Scale data

	Pre-Course	Post-Course
Mean±SD	70.0±11.1	75.9±13.0
P value	0.09	

Discussion

In this pilot experience of developing and executing an IPE course focused on preparing students for team-based practice with vulnerable individuals, faculty educators set out focusing on the students and student learning outcomes. However, as the team of faculty reflected back on the experience in preparation for future offerings with a larger class size, it became apparent that the structure of the faculty team is a critical component to the success of such IPE ventures. As the authors engaged in reflection considering lessons learned, the need to develop and maintain inter-professional cultural competence was discussed and identified as a foundation for success (6). The process of engaging and developing inter-professional cultural competence seems especially true when many professional and institutional barriers exist and collaboration is not a norm. As presented here, there exists an opportunity for inter-professional teams of educators to foster and maintain inter-professional cultural competence. When this process is successful, educators can design significant IPE learning experiences for students. The faculty team can also role model to students the inter-professional cultural competence needed for collaborative care as identified in the mnemonic IDEA.

Furthermore, there remains a significant need for health professions students to gain proficiency in both team skills and preparation for vulnerable patients and populations (9). Integrating team skills with knowledge of how to effectively serve the underserved can prepare a health professional with the aptitude to practice in many health care arenas and address complex issues seen in patient care. Further exploration into the impact of IPE with vulnerable populations is needed. This article also highlights the importance of the passion and compassion of inter-professional faculty to cultivate and devise such complex IPE experiences and the growth needed for such a team when engaging in this type of innovative pedagogy. It further demonstrates that even when facing significant professional and institutional barriers, a passion for social justice and helping those who are vulnerable will prevail. IPE experiences with vulnerable populations will require strong faculty development and institutional support to be successful. But it also cannot be ignored that human nature and care for others remains a critical piece to developing inter-professional cultural competence among faculty which can, in turn, be passed onto students.

References

[1] Inter-professional Education Collaborative. Core competencies for inter-professional collaborative practice: Report of an expert panel. Washington, DC: Inter-professional Education Collaborative, 2011.

[2] Sargeant J, Loney E, Murphy G. Effective inter-professional teams: "contact is not enough" to build a team. J Contin Educ Health Prof 2008;28(4):228-34.

[3] Reeves, S, Zwarenstein, M, Goldman, J, Barr, H, Freeth, D, Koppell, I, et al. The effectiveness of inter-professional education: Key findings from a new systematic review. J Interprof Care 2010;24:230-41.

[4] Hammick, M. Inter-professional education: evidence from the past to guide the future. Med Teacher 2000;22:461-7.

[5] Zorek, J, Raehl C. Inter-professional education accreditation standards in the USA: A comparative analysis. J Interprof Care 2013;27:123-30.

[6] Pecukonis E, Doyle O, Bliss DL. Reducing barriers to inter-professional training: Promoting inter-professional cultural competence. J Interprof Care. 2008;22(4):417-28.

[7] Steinert, Y. Learning together to teach together: inter-professional education and faculty development. J Interprof Care 2005;19:60-75.

[8] Oandasan, I, Reeves, S. Key elements for inter-professional education. Part 1: The learner, the educator and the learning context. J Interprof Care 2005;19:21-38.

[9] Dow A, Blue A, Konrad SC, Earnest M, Reeves S. The moving target: outcomes of inter-professional education. J Interprof Care 2013;27(5):353-5.

[10] Brach, C, Fraserirector, I. Can cultural competency reduce racial and ethnic health disparities? A review and conceptual model. Med Care Res Rev 2000;57:181-217.

[11] Andrulis, DP, Brach, C. Integrating literacy, culture, and language to improve health care quality for diverse populations. Am J Health Behav 2007;31:S122-33.

[12] Eamon, MK. Empowering Vulnerable Populations. Chicago, Illinois: Lyceum Books, 2008.

[13] Royeen CB, Jensen GM, Harvan RA. Leadership in inter-professional health education and practice. Boston, MA: Jones Bartlett, 2011.

[14] Moskowitz D, Glasco J, Johnson B, Wang G. Students in the community: an inter-professional student-run free clinic. J Interprof Care 2006;20(3):254-9.

[15] Bridges DR, Davidson RA, Odegard PS, Maki IV, Tomkowiak J. Inter-professional collaboration: three best practice models of inter-professional education. Med Educ Online 2011;16. doi:10.3402/meo.v16i0.6035

[16] Toner JA, Ferguson KD, Sokal RD. Continuing inter-professional education in geriatrics and gerontology in medically underserved areas. J Contin Educ Health Prof 2009;29(3):157-60.

[17] Hall, P. Inter-professional teamwork: Professional cultures as barriers. J Interprof Care 2005;19:188-96.

[18] Gilbert, JH. Inter-professional learning and higher education structural barriers. J Interprof Care 2005;19:87-106.

[19] Xyrichis, A, Lowton, K. What fosters or prevents inter-professional teamworking in primary and community care? A literature review. Int J Nurs Stud 2008;45:140-53.

[20] Lindqvist, SM, Reeves, S. Facilitators' perceptions of delivering inter-professional education: a qualitative study. Med Teacher 2007;29:403-5.

[21] Grymonpre, R, van Ineveld, C, Nelson, M, Jensen, F, De Jaeger, A, Sullivan, T, et al. See it – Do it – Learn it: Learning inter-professional collaboration in the clinical context. J Res Interprof Pract Educ 2008;1(2):127-144.

[22] Miller, BK, Ishler, JK The rural elderly assessment project: A model for interdisciplinary team training. Occupat Ther Healthcare 2001;15:13-34

[23] Coster, S, Norman, I, Murrells, T, Kitchen, S, Meerabeau, E., Sooboodoo, E et al. Inter-professional attitudes amongst undergraduate students in the health professions: A longitudinal questionnaire survey. Int J Nurs Stud 2008;45:1667-81.

Section two: Inter-professional case examples

In: Public Health
Editors: Rosemary M. Caron and Joav Merrick

ISBN: 978-1-63321-569-6

Chapter 5

A financial education program and health of single, low-income women and their children

Kathleen A Packard*[*]*, PharmD*[2]*, Julie C Kalkowski, MSW*[1]*,
Nicole D White, PharmD*[2]*, Ann M Ryan-Haddad, PharmD*[2]*,
Lisa L Black, DPT*[2]*, Kathleen A Flecky, OTD*[2]*,
Jennifer A Furze, DPT*[2]*, Lorraine M Rusch, PhD*[3]
and Yongyue Qi, MS*[2]

[1]Financial Hope Collaborative, Creighton University College of Business Administration, Omaha, Nebraska, US

[2]School of Pharmacy and Health Professions, Creighton University, Omaha, Nebraska, US

[3]School of Nursing, Creighton University, Omaha, Nebraska, US

Literature suggests an association between poverty, gender, and health. The Financial Success Program (FSP) provides financial education and support to low-income, single mothers. This study assessed the effect of the FSP on health and quality of life in participants and their children. From 2011-2012, 36 women and 28 children were enrolled. Indicators of health and quality of life were assessed pre-and post-year-long intervention. In addition to improvements in financial outcomes, participants demonstrated a significant reduction in fast food consumption and significant improvements in hopefulness and quality of life. Over 30% of mothers experienced weight loss, 52% a reduction in BMI, and 41% a reduction in body fat percentage. Many children experienced reductions in BMI and BMI percentile. In this chapter we report on the health effect of financial education in low-income single mothers. When designing multifaceted community-based cardiovascular risk reduction programs, financial stress should be addressed through education.

[*] Correspondence: Kathleen A. Packard, PharmD, MS, BCPS, Associate Professor of Pharmacy Practice, School of Pharmacy and Health Professions, Creighton University, 2500 California Plaza, Omaha, Nebraska, United States. E-mail: kpackard@creighton.edu.

Introduction

In 2012, 40% of households reported living paycheck to paycheck, a trend more common in women than men, 36% versus 44% (1). The same survey demonstrated that 20% of workers were unable to make ends meet, which can lead to significant financial and socioeconomic stress. Increases in perceived life stress and impairments in well-being have been documented in individuals enduring financial strain (2-6).

Persons under stress can be more socially isolated and report elevated depressive and psychosomatic symptoms (7). They also engage in unhealthy behaviors such as smoking, alcohol consumption, overspending, and poor diet and exercise (8). This has been recently explained by the limited-resource model of self-control (8). Because the poor have less money, food, and expendable time, they are challenged to control behavior and resist urges more than others which exhaust self-control resources. Over time, people under stress are at a greater risk for chronic illness, particularly cardiovascular disease. Financial stress was shown to predict myocardial infarction and cardiac death in women in the Framingham Study and has been associated with coronary heart disease (9,10).

While lifestyle factors can contribute to the development of chronic illness, lower socioeconomic status is also associated with biologic risk factors including hyperlipidemia, obesity, metabolic syndrome, diabetes, elevations in fibrinogen, cardiac rhythm abnormalities, and procoagulant blood profiles (11-13). Many researchers have postulated that the link between stress and poor health outcomes is sustained activation of autonomic and neuroendocrine responses (14). Increased activation of the hypothalamic-pituitary-adrenal axis leading to increased levels of cortisol is a major component of the stress pathway. Chronic cortisol elevations may contribute to insulin resistance, muscle atrophy, diabetes, abdominal fat, immune impairment, and hypertension (7,15). Furthermore, increased sympathetic nervous system activity, specifically elevations in catecholamines, epinephrine and norepinephrine, has been shown in those of lower socioeconomic status (16). Poverty, low socioeconomic status, and financial stress can also affect health outcomes in children. Financial stress during childhood has been associated with increased childhood obesity and the development of diabetes and cardiovascular disease later in life (17-20).

The Financial Success Program (FSP), founded in 2010 at Creighton University, was developed to explore which financial education program components are most effective in creating behavior change for low-income single mothers. The FSP focuses on three core components: an outstanding trainer, one-on-one financial coaching, and an easy to use money management system. The program serves women in the Omaha, Nebraska metropolitan area who are predominantly African American. Participants have significantly more cardiovascular risk factors than other women in Nebraska including obesity, smoking, diminished exercise, hypertension, and diabetes (21).

During the FSP, participants meet weekly for nine weeks followed by monthly group meetings for one year. Participants are also assigned a coach for long-term financial advice. Based on anecdotally-reported positive health changes in prior graduates of the FSP, this study was designed to evaluate the effect of the FSP on cardiovascular risk health indicators and financial outcomes in participants and their children. Figure 1 depicts a conceptual model to describe the relationship between financial education and health indicators. To date, there are no published studies assessing the effect of financial education interventions on health indicators.

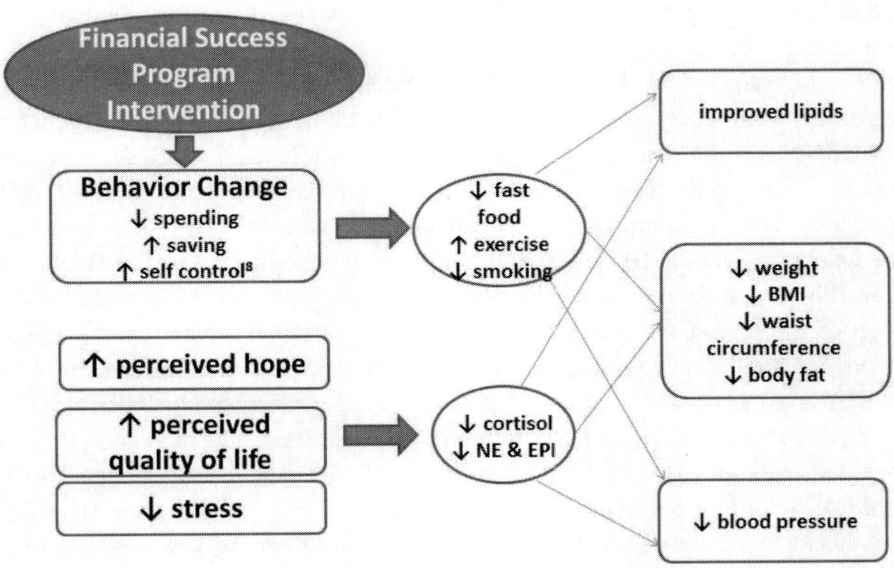

Figure 1. Conceptual Model of the Relationship between the FSP and Health Indicators.

Our study

This study was approved by the Creighton University Institutional Review Board (#11-16171). All participants provided written informed consent/assent as applicable. The study was registered on clinicaltrials.gov as "Impact of a Financial Success Education Program in Women and Children", NCT01409291, on July 29, 2011.

All women enrolled in the FSP between September 2011 and May 2012 were approached for participation in the study. To qualify for the FSP, women were 19 years or older and currently employed. Women were excluded from the FSP if they were abusing alcohol or recreational drugs and were excluded from the study if they were pregnant or planning to become pregnant. Children between 3 and 18 years were also approached for participation in the study. A total of 36 women and 28 children chose to participate in the year-long study.

The FSP curriculum has been described in depth in another publication (22). Prior to the education intervention, baseline demographic, clinical, financial, and questionnaire data were obtained from participants and their children. The same data were collected at the one-year follow-up visit post-intervention. Demographic parameters collected in mothers included age, race, annual household income, education, smoking status, marital status, number of children, type of healthcare insurance, occupational status, frequency of exercise, consumption of fast food, medications, and chronic illnesses.

Due to the outcome of cardiovascular risk reduction, the presence of certain chronic illnesses were defined as follows: hypertension as self-reported, a systolic blood pressure greater $\geq$ 140 mmHg, a diastolic blood pressure $\geq$ 90 mmHg, or use of an antihypertensive drug; diabetes as self-reported, a hemoglobin A1C $\geq$ 6.5%, or use of an anti-diabetic medication; and hyperlipidemia as either self-reported, a total cholesterol $\geq$ 200 mg/dl, or use of a cholesterol-lowering medication. Demographic parameters collected in children included age, race, gender, smoking status, chronic illnesses, frequency of exercise, and consumption of fast food.

Clinical data collected in mothers included blood pressure, weight, body mass index (BMI), waist circumference, hemoglobin A1C, total cholesterol, low density lipoprotein cholesterol (LDL-C), high density lipoprotein cholesterol (HDL-C), triglycerides, and body fat percentage. Clinical data collected in children included blood pressure, weight, BMI, BMI percentile, and waist circumference. Blood pressure was measured in mothers and children three times using an Omron 10 Series digital sphygmomanometer (Omron Healthcare Co, Lake Forest, Illinois) on the dominant arm five minutes apart, at least 15 minutes after arrival. The average of three readings was recorded while the participant was seated. Weight was measured on a digital scale with shoes and coats off. BMI was calculated as weight in kg/(height in meters)^2. Waist circumference was measured by the same operator at both visits. A flexible tape measure was placed on the top of the iliac crest and recorded to the nearest half inch upon patient exhalation. A non-fasting lipid panel was obtained using the CholestechLDX ™ point of care device (Cholestech, Hayward, California) using reflectance photometry. Hands were cleaned with alcohol and the target finger was wiped with an alcohol pad. Enough blood to fill a capillary tube (approximately 5-10 drops) was obtained via fingerstick and was placed into the test cassette by depressing the plunger and inserted into the CholestechLDX ™ machine. Hemoglobin A1C was measured using a DCA Vantage™ Analyzer (Siemans, Deerfield, Illinois). The same fingerstick for the lipid panel was used to obtain the hemoglobin A1C sample. A bioelectrical impedance machine, Omron Model HBF-306C Fat Loss Monitor, (Omron Healthcare Inc., Bannockburn, Illinois) was used to measure body fat percentage.

Qualitative outcomes captured from the mothers at both visits included perceived hopefulness as measured by the Trait Hope Scale (23). Scores range from 8-64, with higher scores indicating more hopefulness. Quality of life was measured with the World Health Organization Quality of Life (WHOQOL)–BREF survey (24). Financial competency and financial health were measured with questions to capture objective and subjective data. For subjective questions, participants provided answers on a Likert Scale (1-5) coded as ordinal data for statistical analysis (1=Never, 2=Seldom, 3=Sometimes, 4=Frequently, 5=Always).

Data analysis

Statistical analyses were performed using SPSS Statistics version 20 (IBM Corporation, Somers, New York). Descriptive statistics were used to describe most baseline demographics. Mean and standard deviations were calculated for continuous variables while a number and a percentage are reported for categorical variables. Comparisons of outcomes pre- and post-intervention were conducted. Dichotomous variables were compared using McNemar's test. A Student's paired, two-tailed t test was used to compare continuous variables. A p value less than 0.05 was considered statistically significant. Data from subjective financial health survey questions (Likert Scale) were compared pre- and post-intervention using non-parametric Wilcoxon Signed Ranks test.

Findings

From September 2011 through May 2012, 36 women and 28 children were enrolled in the study. Follow-up continued through May 2013 with 29 women and 19 children returning for the final visit. Most women and children were African American (59% and 52%, respectively) with a mean annual income of $31,214±$13,726 (Tables 1 and 2). The mean age was 35.8±6.1 years for mothers and 7.0±2.8 years for children. Interestingly, 95% of women were college educated and 66% were never married. Participants had contact with their financial coach an average of 6.9 times per month, either by phone, email, or face to face.

Table 1. Baseline Demographics in Mothers

Mean Age (years)	35.8 ± 6.1
Race	African American 17 (59%), White 11 (38%), Asian 1 (3%)
Mean Annual Household Income (dollars)	$31,214 ± $13,726
Education	College Graduate 14 (48%), Some College 13 (45%), Some High School 1 (3%), High School Graduate 1 (3%)
Marital Status	Never Married 19 (66%), Divorced 6 (21%), Separated 3 (10%), Married 1 (3%)
Mean Number of Children Living with Mother	1.83 ± 1.20

Table 2. Baseline Demographics in Children

Mean Age (years)	7.0 ± 2.8
Gender	Female 11 (58%), Male 8 (42%)
Race	African American 10 (52%), Mixed Race 6 (31%), White 3 (17%)

Financial outcomes

At the end of one year, participants experienced a significant reduction in the mean annual number of overdrawn bank accounts (pre-2.1±2.1, post-1.1±1.7, p=.009), annual shut off notices (pre-2.4±2.2, post-1.0±1.2, p=.003), annual pay day lender utilization (pre-1.4±2.3, post-0.3±0.7, p=.01), and annual bills paid late (pre-3.7±1.9, post-1.8±1.8, p<.0005) (Figure 2). Participants also experienced significant improvements in mean annual medical care access and reductions in annual community agency use.

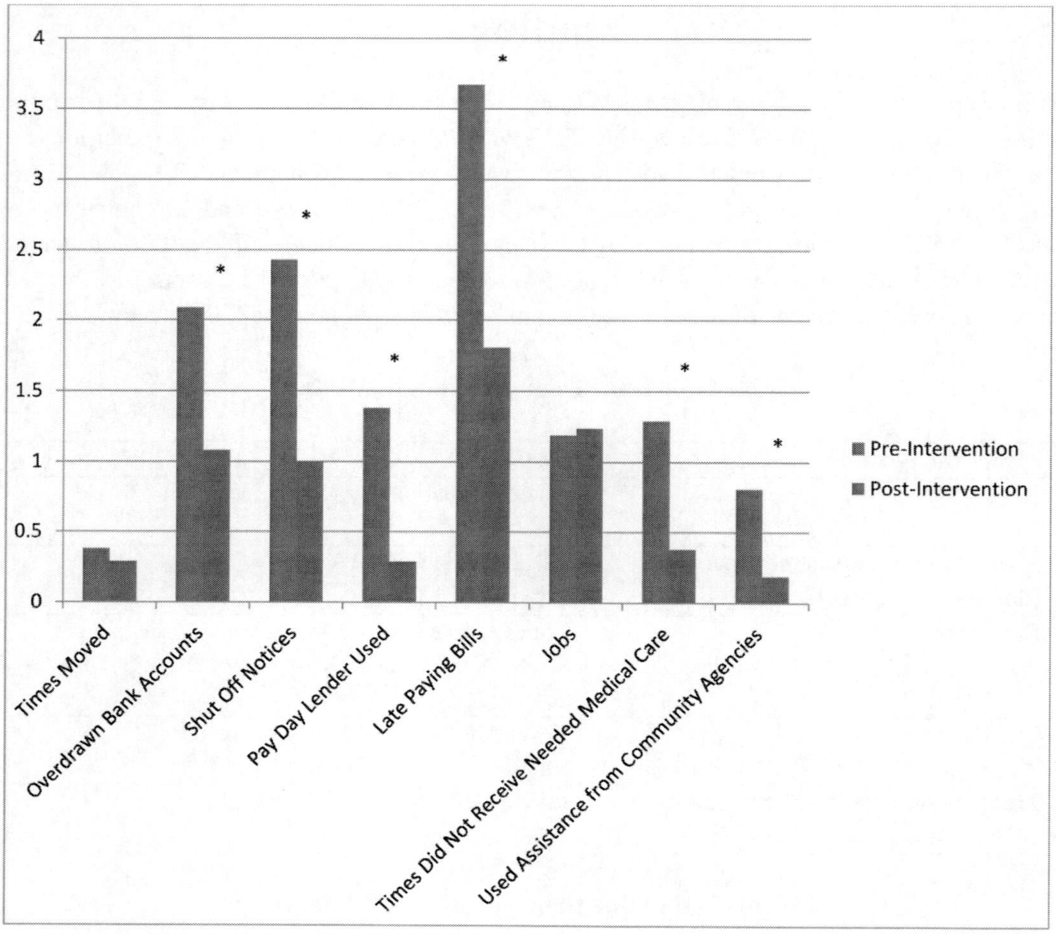

*P<0.05

Figure 2. Objective Financial Health Data Pre- and Post-Intervention (n=21) Mean Number of Occurrences Reported in Previous Year.

Survey data also indicated that the participants significantly reduced their financial stress including lost sleep over money, fighting with their partner about money, and allowing financial stress to affect health, relationships, and their ability to work (Figure 3).

Health indicators

There were no significant changes in the rate of chronic illness after the year-long intervention in women (Table 3). At baseline, 41% of women had hypertension, 24% were smokers, 14% had diabetes, 17% had hyperlipidemia, and 17% reported depression. Though not significant, the rate of hypertension was reduced from 41% to 34% post-intervention. There were also no significant changes in the use of medications in women (Table 4).

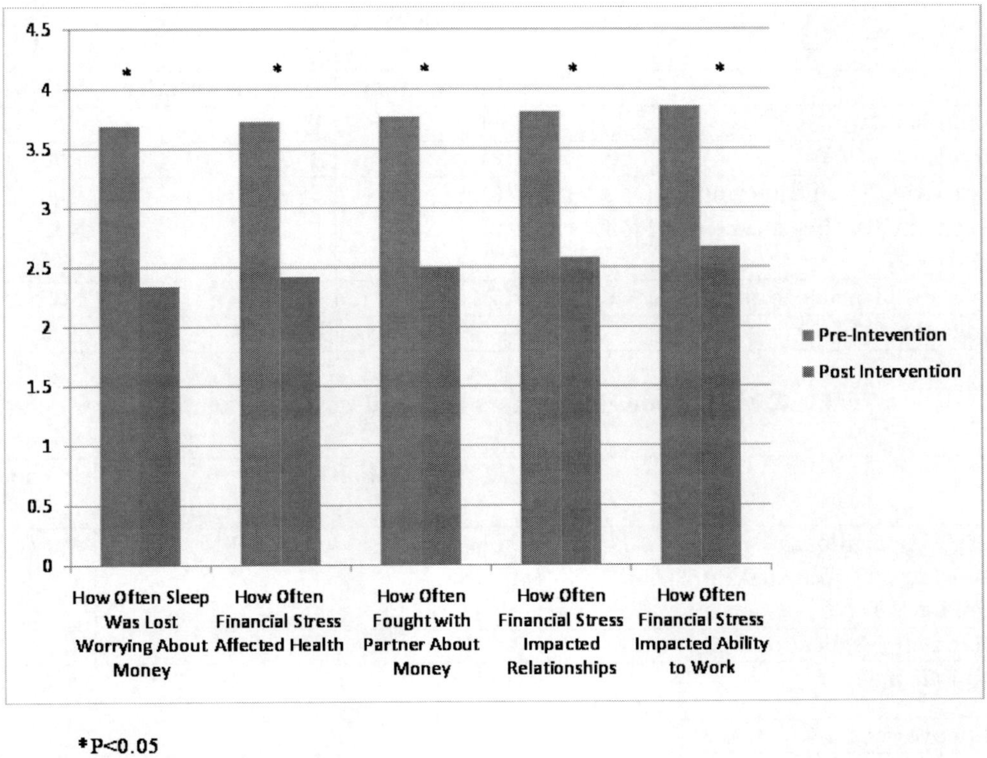

Figure 3. Subjective Financial Health Data Pre- and Post-Intervention (n=21)
Answers Provided on Likert Scale on Occurrence in Previous Year (1=Never, 2=Seldom, 3=Sometimes, 4=Frequently, 5=Always).

Table 3. Chronic Illness in Mothers Pre- and Post-Intervention

	Pre-Intervention	Post-Intervention	P value
Allergies n(%)	2 (7%)	1 (3%)	1.00
Angina n(%)	0	1 (3%)	NA
Anxiety n(%)	4 (14%)	4 (14%)	1.00
Asthma n(%)	3 (10%)	2 (7%)	1.00
Attention Deficit Hyperactivity Disorder n(%)	1 (3%)	1 (3%)	1.00
Bipolar Disorder n(%)	2 (7%)	2 (7%)	1.00
Chrohn's Disease/Irritable Bowel Disease n(%)	1 (3%)	2 (7%)	1.00
Depression n(%)	5 (17%)	4 (14%)	1.00
Type II Diabetes n(%)	4 (14%)	4 (14%)	1.00
Gastroesophageal Reflux Disease n(%)	5 (17%)	5 (17%)	1.00
Headaches/Migraines n(%)	5 (17%)	4 (14%)	1.00
Hyperlipidemia n(%)	5 (17%)	6 (21%)	1.00
Hypertension n(%)	12 (41%)	10 (34%)	0.73

Table 3. (Continued)

	Pre-Intervention	Post-Intervention	P value
Insomnia n(%)	1 (3%)	0	NA
Narcolepsy n(%)	1 (3%)	1 (3%)	1.00
Obstructive Sleep Apnea n(%)	2 (7%)	2 (7%)	1.00
Osteoarthritis/Musculoskeletal Pain n(%)	2 (7%)	0	NA
Polycystic Ovarian Syndrome n(%)	1 (3%)	1 (3%)	1.00
Smokers n(%)	7 (24%)	6 (21%)	1.00

Table 4. Medications in Mothers Pre- and Post-Intervention

	Pre-Intervention	Post-Intervention	P Value
Allergy Medication: Antihistamine/Decongestant/Nasal Steroid n(%)	7 (24%)	7 (24%)	1.00
Antianxiety Medication n(%)	2 (7%)	3 (10%)	1.00
Antibiotic n(%)	1 (3%)	1 (3%)	1.00
Antidepressant n(%)	3 (10%)	3 (10%)	1.00
Antihypertensive n(%)	4 (14%)	5 (17%)	1.00
Antiviral n(%)	1 (3%)	0	NA
Asthma Medication n(%)	1 (3%)	1 (3%)	1.00
Diabetes Medication n(%)	3 (10%)	3 (10%)	1.00
Gastroesophageal Reflux Disease Medication n(%)	3 (10%)	4 (14%)	1.00
Headache/Migraine Medication n(%)	1 (3%)	1 (3%)	1.00
Multivitamin n(%)	7 (24%)	5 (17%)	0.73
Non-Steroidal Anti-Inflammatory or Acetaminophen n(%)	7 (24%)	6 (21%)	1.00
Opioid Analgesic n(%)	1 (3%)	0	NA
Oral Contraceptive n(%)	5 (17%)	4 (14%)	1.00
Psychostimulant n(%)	1 (3%)	2 (7%)	1.00
Sleep Aid n(%)	0	1 (3%)	NA

There were significant reductions in weekly fast food consumption in both women and children; 2.4$\pm$1.7 weekly meals reduced to 1.5$\pm$1.1 , p=.010 and 1.9$\pm$1.4 weekly meals reduced to 1.4$\pm$1.3, p=.03 for women and children, respectively (Tables 5 and 6). There were also trends towards increased exercise in mothers, 120.0$\pm$237.0 weekly minutes pre-intervention and 184.2$\pm$404.2 minutes post-intervention, p=.35.

Table 5. Lifestyle Modifications in Mothers Pre- and Post-Intervention

	Pre-Intervention	Post-Intervention	P Value
Mean Minutes of Exercise per Week	120.0 ± 237.0	184.2 ± 404.2	0.35
Mean Weekly Fast Food Consumption	2.4 ± 1.7	1.5 ± 1.1	0.010*

*P<0.05

Table 6. Lifestyle Modifications in Children Pre- and Post-Intervention

	Pre-Intervention	Post -Intervention	P value
Mean Minutes of Exercise per Week	404.5 ± 319.6	350.3 ± 246.8	0.38
Mean Weekly Fast Food Consumption	1.9 ± 1.4	1.4 ± 1.3	0.03*

There were no significant changes in any of the mean cardiovascular risk factor or biometric data (Table 7) for mothers. While there was no difference in the mean change in weight, nine of the women (31%) lost weight, between 6 and 28 pounds. Fifteen women (52%) experienced a BMI reduction, ten (34%) experienced a waist circumference reduction, and 12 (41%) experienced a body fat percentage reduction.

Table 7. Cardiovascular Risk Factors in Mothers Pre- and Post-Intervention

	Pre-Intervention	Post-Intervention	P Value
Mean Systolic Blood Pressure (mmHg)	117.0 ± 15.5	118.4 ± 15.5	0.47
Mean Diastolic Blood Pressure (mmHg)	81.5 ± 13.1	82.3 ± 12.0	0.72
Mean Weight (pounds)	198.2 ± 58.5	197.3 ± 56.8	0.71
Mean Body Mass Index	33.4 ± 9.6	33.3 ± 8.6	0.81
Mean Waist Circumference (inches)	39.5 ± 7.2	40.0 ± 6.7	0.44
Mean Body Fat %	36.0 ± 8.8	37.2 ± 7.2	0.17
Mean Hemoglobin A1C %	5.7 ± 0.37	5.8 ± 0.80	0.25
Mean Total Cholesterol mg/dl	179.8 ± 29.3	173.4 ± 31.5	0.39
Mean Low-Density Lipoprotein Cholesterol mg/dl	93.0 ± 26.0	96.3 ± 30.4	0.58
Mean High-Density Lipoprotein Cholesterol mg/dl	53.1 ± 15.1	49.4 ± 12.8	0.11
Mean Triglycerides mg/dl	147.0 ± 75.0	147.2 ± 110.7	0.08

Other than expected increases in normal growth, there were no significant changes in cardiovascular risk data for children (Table 8). While there were no significant differences in the mean change in BMI, eight children (42%) experienced a BMI reduction and six (32%) experienced a BMI percentile reduction.

Table 8. Cardiovascular Risk Factors in Children Pre- and Post-Intervention

	Pre-Intervention	Post-Intervention	P Value
Mean Body Mass Index	18.4 ± 4.6	19.3 ± 5.6	0.05
Mean Body Mass Index Percentile	63.2% ± 30.1%	61.0% ± 33.1%	0.57
Mean Waist Circumference (inches)	25.1 ± 5.2	26.4 ± 5.2	0.001*
Mean Height (inches)	50.6 ± 6.5	53.2 ± 6.3	<0.0001*
Mean Weight (pounds)	71.1 ± 34.7	82.6 ± 41.6	<0.0001*
Mean Systolic Blood Pressure (mmHg)	95.8 ± 9.1	93.0 ± 9.1	0.30
Mean Diastolic Blood Pressure (mmHg)	62.7 ± 11.0	59.1 ± 8.0	0.20

*P<0.05

Quality of life in mothers improved for all domains assessed (Table 9). This was statistically significant for domain 1, physical health (pre-21.2±3.0 and post-23.3±3.0, p=.001) and domain 4, environment (pre-26.6±4.8 and post-30.1±5.6, p<.001). Likewise, Trait Hope Scale scores significantly improved for mothers (pre-48.7±7.9 and post-52.7±8.5, p=.01)

Table 9. World Health Organization Quality of Life-BREF Raw Score and Trait Hope Scale Score in Women Pre- and Post-Intervention

	Pre-Intervention	Post-Intervention	P Value
Mean Domain 1 Physical Health	21.2 ± 3.0	23.3 ± 3.0	0.001*
Mean Domain 2 Psychological	19.8 ± 3.2	20.8 ± 3.2	0.10
Mean Domain 3 Social Relationships	10.0 ± 2.5	10.8 ± 2.9	0.20
Mean Domain 4 Environment	26.6 ± 4.8	30.1 ± 5.6	<0.001*
Mean Trait Hope Scale Score	48.7 ± 7.9	52.7 ± 8.5	0.01*

*P<0.05

Discussion

Financial education through the FSP led to significant improvements in measurements of financial outcomes including reductions in overdrawn bank accounts, reductions in shut off notices, reductions in pay day lender use, reductions in late bill payments, improvements in health care access, and reductions in community agency use. These behavior changes also improved social and physical well-being including significant reductions in lost sleep over money, reductions in fighting with their partner about money, and less effect of financial stress on health, relationships, and ability to work.

This is the first study to demonstrate that a financial education program can affect physical health. Both women and children significantly reduced their consumption of fast food. This was probably due to the FSP emphasis of the negative effect of eating out not only on physical health but on finances. There were also trends towards increased weekly exercise in mothers, but not the children. Self-reporting of exercise in children was highly variable and anecdotally, mothers reported difficulty in estimating exercise, especially in their younger, more active children. Mothers were uncertain of physical activities their children engaged in during school-based physical education classes, recess, or after-school programs.

While there were no significant changes in any of the mean cardiovascular risk or biometric data for mothers, many of the women experienced weight loss and reductions in BMI, waist circumference, and body fat percentage. This is important as it has been shown in cohorts from the Nurses' Health Studies I and II that women gain, on average, approximately 3.35 pounds every four years (25). Data from the Behavioral Risk Factor Surveillance System similarly showed that women gain 0.3 kg or 0.7 pounds per year (26). The fact that so many women in this study lost weight needs to be further explored. Similarly, for children, while there were no significant differences in the mean change in BMI, many experienced a reduction in BMI and BMI percentile.

There are reasons why participants may not have experienced significant changes in blood pressure, lipid panels, hemoglobin A1C, and biometric parameters. First, the primary objective of the FSP is to improve immediate financial outcomes. There are only limited direct health interventions embedded within the program. Those that are implemented such as reduction of fast food or changing medications to generic or "$4 list" have a direct effect on finances and were significantly improved. Therefore, expansion of the program to integrate direct health interventions is planned for the future.

Second, a one year follow-up duration may not have been adequate for all participants to implement lifestyle changes necessary to reduce cardiovascular risk. While many of the women experienced weight loss and positive changes in their BMI, body fat percentage, and waist circumference, others remained the same or gained weight. Anecdotally, some women reported that one year was just enough time to become financially secure and now they could begin to focus on reducing cardiovascular risk. Therefore, investigators intend to follow participants for one more year to assess for further changes and determine sustainability of change.

A recent study in socially disadvantaged women assessing a two-year community-based primary prevention program to reduce cardiovascular risk supports this timeline to some degree (27). While the program was multi-faceted in that it encompassed exercise, nutrition, psychological and relaxation, it did not reportedly provide financial education. The findings indicated a significant decrease in metabolic syndrome at year one (64.7% versus 34.9%, $p=.01$) and even more at year two (28.2%, $p<.001$), driven by significant reductions in blood pressure and increases in HDL-C. Hemoglobin A1C was also further improved after two years of follow-up (6% at year one, 5.85% at year two ($p=.87$) and 5.8% at year three ($p<.01$)). Unlike the FSP, this study did not achieve significant reductions in fast food consumption, perhaps because it was not linked to a financial benefit. Similar to the FSP, this study did not achieve significant reductions in waist circumference or triglycerides.

FSP participants experienced statistically significant improvements in perceived hope and also quality of life for the domains of physical health and environment, with the most pronounced increase in environment. In the WHO QOL-BREF, the environment domain includes financial resources, information and skills, recreation and leisure, home environment, access to health and social care, physical safety and security, physical environment, and transport. Improvements in these domains are therefore consistent with other study results demonstrating improvement in financial and health indicators. In a recent study, perceived well-being was shown to be a strong predictor of health care outcomes including hospital admissions, emergency room visits, and health care costs (28). Each point increase in well-being was associated with a 1% reduction in health care costs and those with low scores had a 2.7 times increase in annual expenditures compared with those having high scores. Therefore, future research should be conducted to ascertain whether the FSP also reduces health care costs.

Limitations

Several important limitations of this study should be mentioned. Recruitment for the FSP is predominantly through word of mouth and there is an ongoing waiting list to enter the program. Therefore, these women may have been more motivated to change than other women in the general population. There is no control group that did not receive the financial intervention. While this is an important limitation, due to the wait list to enter the program, investigators did not feel it would be ethical to randomize a control group from this sample. Likewise, although these women are low-income, their mean income was $31,214±$13,726 and 95% of them had some college education or were college graduates. In 2012, the poverty threshold for a family of four was $23,050 (29). Only 34% of the women in this study fell below the poverty line. Therefore, it may be inappropriate to extrapolate these data to women living below the poverty line or those with less education. Also, because the study visits occurred in the evening after work, most were in a non-fasting state. This could have affected the lipid panel results. Likewise, fluid intake was not assessed and this can affect body fat percentage readings from the bioelectrical impedance machine. However, because the visits occurred at the same time both pre- and post-intervention, it is expected that these variables were equally distributed between both visits. Finally, the FSP also limits its enrollment in order to optimize group interactions. The small sample size restricts the generalizability of the results.

Conclusion

This study is the first to report the positive effect of a financial education program in low-income single women on health indicators. In this high risk population, it was found that a year-long financial education intervention led to significant reductions in fast food consumption, improvements in perceived hope and quality of life. While there were no significant changes in any of the mean cardiovascular risk factor or biometric data for mothers, many of the women experienced weight loss and reductions in BMI, waist circumference, and body fat percentage. Similarly, for children, while there were no significant differences in the mean change in BMI, many experienced a reduction in BMI and BMI percentile.

Multifaceted community-based cardiovascular risk reduction programs are important. When designing such interventions, financial stress, which is often a major barrier for single low-income women to adopt a healthy lifestyle, should be addressed through education.

Further research needs to be conducted to determine the critical components of such programs and optimal follow-up.

Acknowledgments

This work was supported by funding from the Creighton University Dr. George F. Haddix President's Faculty Research Fund, the Ruth and William Scott Family Foundation, Sherwood Foundation, Weitz Funds, and United Way of the Midlands. The authors would like to thank Kate Martens Stricklett and Ronna Sears-Fritz for their assistance and support throughout the investigation. None of the authors have any current or past commercial associations that may pose a conflict of interest. No financial disclosures were reported by the authors of this paper.

References

[1] Careerbuilder.com. Percentage of U.S. workers living paycheck to paycheck reaches recession-era low, finds careerbuilder survey. Accessed 2013 July 09. URL: http://www.careerbuilder.com/share/aboutus/pressreleasesdetail.aspx?sd=8%2F15%2F2012&id=pr711&ed=12%2F31%2F2012.

[2] Kessler RC, Cleary PD. Social class and psychological distress. Am Social Rev 1980;45:463-78.

[3] Seeman TE, Crimmins E. Social environment effects on health and aging: integrating epidemiologic and demographic approaches and perspectives. Ann NY Acad Sci 2001;954:88-117.

[4] Turner RJ, Wheaton B, Lloyd DA. The epidemiology of social stress. Am Social Rev 1995;60:104-25.

[5] Garcia MC, de Souza A, Bella GP et al. Salivary cortisol levels in Brazilian citizens of distinct socioeconomic and cultural levels. Ann NY Acad Sci 2008;1148:504-8.

[6] Dettenborn L, Tietze A, Bruckner F, et al. Higher cortisol content in hair among long-term unemployed individuals compared to controls. Psychoneuroendocrinology 2010;35(9):1404-9.

[7] Grossi G, Perski A, Lundberg U, et al. Associations between financial strain and the diurnal salivary cortisol secretion of long-term unemployed individuals. Integr Physiol Behav Sci 2001;36:205-19.

[8] Vohs KD. Psychology. The poor's poor mental power. Science 2013;341:969-70.

[9] Eaker ED, Pinsky J, Castelli WP. Myocardial infarction and coronary death among women: psychosocial predictors from a 20-year follow-up of women in the Framingham Study. Am J Epidemiol 1992;135:854-64.

[10] Rosengren A, Hawken S, Ounpuu S, et al. Association of psychosocial risk factors with risk of acute myocardial infarction in 11,119 cases and 13,648 controls from 52 countries (the INTERHEART study): case-control study. Lancet 2004;364:953-62.

[11] Kunz-Ebrecht SR, Kirschbaum C, Steptoe A. Work stress, socioeconomic status and neuroendocrine activation over the working day. Soc Sci Med 2004;58:1523-30.

[12] Steptoe A, Phil D, Brydon L, et al. Changes in financial strain over three years, ambulatory blood pressure, and cortisol response to awakening. Psychosomatic Med 2005;67:281-7.

[13] Ogden CL, Lamb MM, Carroll MD, et al. Obesity and socioeconomic status in adults: United States, 2005-2008. 2010. NCHS Data Brief No. 50; 1-8.

[14] Dowd JB, Goldman N. Do biomarkers of stress mediate the relation between socioeconomic status and health. J Epidemiol Community Health 2006;60:633-39.

[15] Bjorntorp P, Rosemond R. The metabolic syndrome – a neuroendocrine disorder? Br J Nutr 2000;83:49-57.

[16] Janicki-Deverts D, Cohen S, Adler NE, et al. Socioeconomic status is related to urinary catecholamines in the Coronary Artery Risk Development in Young Adults (CARDIA) study. Psychosom Med 2007;69:514-20.

[17] Gundersen C, Mahatmya D, Garasky S, et al. Linking psychosocial stressors and childhood obesity. Obes Rev 2011;12:e54-63.

[18] Chichlowska KL, Rose KM, Diez-Roux AV, et al. Life course socioeconomic conditions and metabolic syndrome in adults: the Atherosclerosis Risk in Communities (ARIC) Study. Ann Epidemiol 2009;19:875-83.

[19] Lidfeldt J, Li TY, Hu FB, et al. A prospective study of childhood and adult socioeconomic status and incidence of type 2 diabetes in women. Am J Epidemiol 2007;165:882-9.

[20] Galobardes B, Smith GD, Lynch JW. Systematic review of the influence of childhood socioeconomic circumstances on risk for cardiovascular disease in adulthood. Ann Epidemiol 2006;16:91-104.

[21] Gillespie N, Packard KA, Kalkowski J, et al. Cardiovascular risk factors of women and children in an urban financial education program. Presented at: Preventive Medicine Annual Meeting. Orlando, (FL), February 2012.

[22] White N, Packard K, Kalkowski J, et al. A novel financial education program in single women of low-income and their children. Int Pub Health J 2013, in Press.

[23] Snyder CR, Harris C, Anderson JR, et al. The will and the ways: development and validation of an individual-differences measure of hope. J Person Soc Psychol 1991;60:570-85.

[24] The WHOQOL Group. Development of the World Health Organization WHOQOL-BREF quality of life assessment. Psychol Med 1998;28:551–8.

[25] Mozaffarian D, Hao T, Rimm EB, et al. Changes in diet and lifestyle and long-term weight gain in women and men. N Engl J Med 2011;363:2392-2404.

[26] Wetmore CM, Mokdad AH. In denial: misperceptions of weight change among adults in the United States. Prev Med 2012;55:93-100.

[27] Gilstrap LG, Malhotra R, Peltier-Saxe D et al. Community-based primary prevention programs decrease the rate of metabolic syndrome among socioeconomically disadvantaged women. J Wom Health 2013;22(4):322-8.

[28] Harrison PL, Pope JE, Coberley CR, et al. Evaluation of the relationship between individual well-being and future health care utilization and cost. Pop Health Manag 2012;15:325-30.

[29] US Department of Health and Human Services. 2012 poverty guidelines. Accessed 2013 July 14. URL: http://aspe.hhs.gov/poverty/12poverty.shtml#thresholds.

In: Public Health
Editors: Rosemary M. Caron and Joav Merrick

ISBN: 978-1-63321-569-6

Chapter 6

Education program for single women of low-income and their children

Nicole White[1*], *Kathleen Packard*[1], *Julie Kalkowski*[2], *Ann Ryan-Haddad*[1], *Kathy Flecky*[1], *Jennifer Furze*[1], *Lori Rusch*[3] *and Lisa Black*[1]

[1]Creighton University School of Pharmacy and Health Professions,
[2]Creighton University College of Business, Financial Hope Collaborative,
[3]Creighton University School of Nursing, Omaha, Nebraska, US

Financial stress is a condition that occurs commonly in the United States, especially in single-mothers and their children. This stress can be a barrier to optimal health and wellness. In an effort to reduce financial stress and improve money management skills in low income, single mother families, the Financial Success Program (FSP) was created. This novel program provides education and support to an underserved population and may also improve the health and well-being of the women and children enrolled. Through a unique inter-professional collaboration, a study was initiated to assess the effect of financial education on health indicators in single-mother families. A thorough discussion of the FSP and inter-professional model will be discussed as a framework for addressing public health needs in a financially stressed population.

Introduction

Traditional risk factors for heart disease include hypertension, hypercholesterolemia, diabetes, obesity, sedentary behavior, smoking and family history (1). Financial stress, however, has also been implicated in cardiovascular disease risk. In the Framingham heart study, financial stress was associated with coronary heart disease and was shown to predict myocardial infarction and cardiac death in women (2,3). Additionally, lower socioeconomic status is

* Corresponding author: Nicole White, PharmD, Assistant Professor, Pharmacy Practice, Creighton University, School of Pharmacy and Health Professions, 2500 California Plaza, Omaha, NE 68178, United States. E-mail: nicolewhite@creighton.edu.

associated with impaired well-being and biologic risk factors for heart disease including hyperlipidemia, metabolic syndrome and diabetes (4-6). Low socioeconomic status and financial stress also have deleterious effects on the health of children, including a greater rate of childhood obesity and subsequent development of diabetes and cardiovascular disease (7-10).

Financial stress is not uncommon. Up to 40% of American households report living paycheck to paycheck (11). Single-mother families may be especially affected by financial strain. A report from 2012 found that 63% of single mother families met the poverty rate in the United States versus a 17% rate of poverty in two-parent families (poverty rate based on the 50% of median income poverty standard) (12). Due to its prevalence and association with poor health outcomes, financial stress presents a novel target for public health interventions, especially in the single-mother family population.

Program history

In an effort to reduce financial stress and improve money management skills in low income, single mother families, the Financial Success Program (FSP) was created. The FSP was initially funded by a grant from the Financial Industry Regulatory Authority (FINRA) Investor Education Foundation in 2010 to explore what financial education program components are most effective in creating behavior change for low income single mothers. The FSP focuses on three core components: an outstanding trainer, financial coaching, and an easy to use money management system.

To be eligible for participation in the FSP, women must be earning a minimum of $12,000 annually, cannot be involved in a domestic violence situation or have an active addiction to alcohol or illicit drugs. They must also be willing to participate in both nine weeks of training and one year of financial coaching. The initial nine-week curriculum was created to address the immediate financial issues in a group of employed women who are struggling financially. The curriculum includes tracking expenses, saving for emergencies, and repairing credit reports. Information on taxes, insurance, predatory lending, legal issues, and the psychology of money are also provided. The nine-week curricular outline is described below (see table 1). The classes are offered once a week for two-three hours in a local community meeting space. Program participants receive free dinner and daycare with each weekly class. Participants are also paired with a financial coach, with whom they work with for a year following the initial classes. Financial coaches review and assess saved receipts, expense tracking forms, pay stubs and credit reports with the women. From this evaluation, spending habits are discussed and women participants make plans for change. Frequency of interaction with the coach is agreed upon by the participant and coach and may vary throughout the year depending on needs. This may include face to face meetings, phone calls, or email interaction. To date 196 women have completed the FSP.

Program methodology

The FSP is a two-phase program. Phase One involves the nine-week didactic curriculum in which women and their children receive a healthy dinner and live interactive educational sessions with an experienced trainer. Free childcare is available during these meetings. Phase Two occurs after graduation from the educational classes and involves one-on-one financial coaching from an assigned FSP representative, as well as monthly graduate follow-up meetings. Coaching is available for one year following the last didactic session and frequency of interaction is determined by the needs of the individual woman. Phase One curriculum is described below (see Table 1).

Inter-professional collaboration

The FSP was developed and is currently directed by individuals affiliated with the Creighton University College of Business Administration in Omaha, Nebraska. Following the first year of program enrollment, the directors noted that cardiovascular risk indicators such as weight and overall well-being were improving in graduates as their financial health improved. Many graduates had either completely given up fast food or had significantly reduced the number of times they ate fast food per week. Based on these preliminary, anecdotal reports, the program directors sought out a partnership with health science colleagues to determine if better finances meant better health for the women and children enrolled in the FSP.

Table 1. Financial Education Curriculum

Session 1	• Introduction to financial support team and program orientation. • Active Learning: Intake form and baseline survey completion (assessing financial state, spending habits and hopefulness), family financial snapshot, financial journaling, asset bingo and receipt saving assignment
Session 2	• Family financial snapshot and psychology of money • Active Learning: Expense tracking
Session 3	• Understanding predatory lending • Active Learning: Expense tracking
Session 4	• Banking and savings, guest speaker • Active learning: expense tracking and assignment to collect paystub for next session
Session 5	• Understanding credit and credit reports and how to increase income without a second job, guest speaker • Active Learning: Learning how to read a credit report, what a credit score means and how your credit score affects your life, and how to fix and/or build credit, introduction to financial coach and expense tracking
Session 6	• Level payment plan, guest speakers from local utility providers • Active Learning: expense tracking and enrolling in the level payment plans for utilities
Session 7	• Legal issues, guest speaker from Legal Aid • Active Learning: Expense tracking, how to read your pay stub and meeting with financial coach
Session 8	• Understanding insurance/retirement, guest speaker
Session 9	• Graduation ceremony • Active Learning: Follow-up survey completion (assessing financial state, spending habits and hopefulness)

The FSP program directors reached out to the Creighton University School of Pharmacy and Health Professions Office of Inter-professional Scholarship, Service and Education (OISSE). The OISSE office is an established structure within Creighton University, designed to organize and promote inter-professional partnerships that offer teaching, scholarship and service opportunities for faculty and students in the health sciences. The OISSE office coordinated the recruitment of health science faculty, students, and residents to collaborate on this project.

This particular inter-professional collaboration is unique in that it bridges social sciences (business administration) with various health care disciplines. Members of the team include a social worker from the college of business administration, three pharmacists, an occupational therapist, a nurse, and three physical therapists.

Based on the hypothesis that decreased financial stress would also lead to cardiovascular risk reduction, an inter-professional study was initiated. The program directors continued to provide the financial education and support within the original structure of the FSP, while the health professional team measured pre and post-intervention biometric and quality of life data to assess for changes in cardiovascular risk and overall well-being. To date, there are no published studies assessing the impact of a financial education intervention on health.

Cardiovascular risk assessment

At the second FSP session, following consent, women are enrolled in the cardiovascular risk assessment study. At this time, baseline demographic, biometric and quality of life data are collected by the team of health care professionals. This data is comprehensive but includes among other measures: age, height, weight, body mass index (BMI), smoking status, cholesterol, hemoglobin A1c (HbA1c), blood pressure, body fat percentage, insurance coverage, income, and quality of life as measured by the World Health Organization (WHO) Quality of Life (QOL) survey (abbreviated version).

During the assessment visit, point of care blood pressure, cholesterol and A1c results are interpreted for each participant and referrals are made when urgent or emergent values are obtained. Additionally, short counseling sessions are completed regarding abnormal lab values and lifestyle behaviors that can be modified to improve biometric data. The risk assessment process is then repeated on the same set of women and children after approximately one year of participation in the FSP.

Not surprisingly, the women enrolled in the FSP were found to have great need for cardiovascular risk reduction. In addition to poor financial status, the women enrolled in FSP also present with significantly more risk factors for cardiovascular disease than other women in Nebraska including greater rates of obesity, tobacco use, diminished exercise, hypertension, and diabetes (see table 2) (13-17). The children of single-mothers enrolled in the FSP were also at increased risk of chronic disease. Compared to 31.5% of children (aged 10-17) in Nebraska, 42.1% of the children assessed in the FSP were overweight or obese (as measured by a BMI>85th percentile for age) (24).

Table 2. Comparison of FSP Participants to Average Women in Nebraska

	Women Enrolled in FSP	Women in Nebraska
Race Caucasian	38%	89.2%[16]
African American	59%	3.3%[16]
No health insurance	6.9%	12.6%[16]
Overweight or Obese BMI (≥25.0)	79.3%	57.3%[14]
Obese BMI (≥30)	58.6%	26.3%[14]
Current Smoker	20.7%	15.1%[13]
Physically Inactive (0 min/week reported)	24.1%	11.6%[15]
Diabetes	13.8%	7.2%[16]
Elevated Cholesterol	34.5%	35.3%[17]
Hypertension	34.5%	25.3%[17]

Public health implications

Due to its prevalence and negative implications on health and well-being, financial stress is a novel target for public health interventions. On a broad level, the FSP, in conjunction with the inter-professional cardiovascular risk assessment, aligns well with several of the Healthy People 2020 goals (see table 3) (18).

Table 3. Healthy People 2020 Goals Addressed by the FSP and Inter-professional Cardiovascular Risk Assessment

Goal	2020 Target
HDS 4 – Increase the proportion of adults who have had their blood pressure measured within the preceding 2 years and can state whether their blood pressure was normal or high	92.6%
HDS 5.1 – Reduce the proportion of adults in the population with hypertension	26.9%
HDS 5.2 – Reduce the proportion of children and adolescents in the population with hypertension	3.2%
HDS 6 - Increase the proportion of adults who have had their blood cholesterol checked within the preceding 5 years	82.1%
HDS 7 - Reduce the proportion of adults with high total blood cholesterol levels	13.5%
HDS 8 - Reduce the mean total blood cholesterol levels among adults	177.9 mg/dl
HDS 11 - Increase the proportion of adults with hypertension who are taking the prescribed medications to lower blood pressure	69.5%
HDS 12 – Increase the proportion of adults with hypertension whose blood pressure is under control	61.2%

HDS: Heart Disease and Stroke.

Additionally, the FSP and inter-professional cardiovascular risk assessment fulfill several of the ten Essential Services of Public Health, as defined by the National Public Health Performance Standards Program (NPHPSP) (19). Specifically, eight Essential Services are demonstrated in the FSP. These include:

1. Monitor health status to identify and solve community health problems
2. Diagnose and investigate health problems and health hazards in the community
3. Inform, educate, and empower people about health issues
4. Mobilize community partnerships and action to identify and solve health problems
5. Link people to needed personal health services and assure the provision of health care when otherwise unavailable
6. Assure competent public and personal health care workforce
7. Evaluate effectiveness, accessibility, and quality of personal and population-based health services
8. Research for new insights and innovative solutions to health problems

The pre/post cardiovascular risk assessments allow the team to monitor the health status and identify health problems affecting single mothers and their children with financial stress (Essential Service 1). The study team has identified that women in the FSP have a higher incidence of obesity, smoking, physical inactivity, diabetes, and hypertension compared to women in Nebraska (Essential Service 2). The FSP program and faculty team members provided health education to empower study participants to implement lifestyle modifications and to seek healthcare to address specific health issues identified in the health assessments (Essential Service 3). The campus-community partnership was successfully developed (with the university infrastructure in place) to recruit health science faculty team members interested in participating with colleagues in business administration to develop a research project assessing the impact of the FSP on women's cardiovascular health (Essential Service 4). On many occasions, team members were able to refer mothers to appropriate low/no cost health clinics for treatment of high blood pressure or diabetes (Essential Service 7). Faculty team members recruited health science students from their own didactic courses or clinical rotations to assist in the health assessments and this provided students with a unique opportunity to work side by side with faculty and develop clinical and social skills to assure competent future health care workforces (Essential Service 8). During the pre/post assessments, faculty team members were able to learn more about accessibility and quality of personal health services and the barriers single mothers with financial stress often encounter (Essential Service 9). The uniqueness of this project will provide new insights into the health effects of financial stress, as well as potentially serve as an innovative model for addressing health issues of single-mother families (Essential Service 10).

Discussion

While many other financial education programs exist, the FSP is unique and highly sought after due to its three core components: an outstanding trainer, financial coaching, and an easy to use money management system. Unlike other financial education programs, where the primary focus is home ownership or small business start-ups, single mothers under financial stress need a plan to help them change their financial behaviors. The FSP focuses on the financial challenges unique to single mothers under financial stress. An outstanding trainer is essential. The trainer for the FSP has significant life experiences, including being a single mother, that complements her skills as a facilitator and allows her to talk about common financial problems faced in this population without evoking a feeling of judgment in the women enrolled.

The second core component of the FSP is the financial coaching. The FSP directors carefully distinguish the word "coach" from "mentor" for this position which ultimately directs the relationship that exists between the coaches and the single-mother participants. The coaches are to work WITH the women in the program to bring about a change in their financial behavior rather than give advice or use confrontation as a financial expert or "mentor". This technique is one example of how motivational interviewing is used by the coaches to elicit financial behavior change (20). Many of the coaches are single-mothers themselves. This attribute allows them to display greater empathy toward the women in the program and support their self-efficacy in making a positive change. Empathy and promotion of self-efficacy are two other key components to motivational interviewing and successful behavior change (20). In addition to motivational interviewing, coaches use various methods of communication to reach the FSP participants. Meetings can occur face to face, over the telephone, through email and via social media. This varied approach ensures that women are being contacted in a way that is convenient and most helpful to them.

The third and final core component of the FSP is an easy to use money management system. Program participants are given an Excel spreadsheet on a jump drive so they can input their expenses. The participants review their expense logs with their financial coaches to identify patterns or areas for improvement. By seeing where their money is being spent, the women realize they have more choices. For many women, it is the first time they feel they have some control in one aspect of their lives. This leads to the realization they also have control in other areas of their lives, including their health and wellness. A sense of internal control (as opposed to being controlled by others or circumstances beyond personal control) has been associated with a perception of being able to impact one's personal health in positive ways (21, 22). Moreover, perception of personal, internal control over stressful events can promote a mindset of less stress and a physiological diminished cortisol response to stressors (23).

For many of the women starting the FSP, being financially stressed takes precedence in their lives which limits their ability to pay attention to information or behaviors related to exercise and nutrition. Making better financial decisions gives women the ability and confidence to focus on issues other than money and empowers them to address the health and wellness of themselves and their family.

Conclusion

Financial stress is a non-traditional risk factor for heart disease and may be a novel target for public health interventions to improve cardiovascular risk and overall well-being. Single-mother families have higher reported rates of poverty than two parent families and endure significantly higher financial strain. The FSP is an innovative program focused on decreasing financial stress and improving money-management skills in low-income single-mother families. The program is also being evaluated for its effect on health and well-being. To date, this is the only published study assessing the impact of a financial education intervention on health. The program and study highlight a unique inter-professional partnership that bridges social sciences (business administration) with health care disciplines (pharmacy, occupational therapy, physical therapy and nursing). The collaboration allows for expert attention to both personal finances and personal health with broad public health implications. Further research will determine whether the program makes a significant impact on the health and well being of the single mother families that participate.

References

[1] DeGoma EM, Knowles JW, Angeli F, Budoff MJ, Rader DJ. The evolution and refinement of traditional risk factors for cardiovascular disease. Cardiol Rev 2012;20(3):118-29.

[2] Eaker ED, Pinsky J, Castelli WP. Myocardial infarction and coronary death among women: psychosocial predictors from a 20-year follow-up of women in eth Framingham Study. Am J Epidemiol 1992;135:854-64.

[3] Rosengren A, Hawken S, Ounpuu S, et al. Association of psychosocial risk factors with risk of acute myocardial infarction in 11,119 cases and 13,648 controls from 52 countries (the INTERHEART study): case-control study. Lancet 2004;364:953-62.

[4] Kunz-Ebrecht SR, Kirschbaum C, Steptoe A. Work stress, socioeconomic status and neuroendocrine activation over the working day. Soc Sci Med 2004;58:1523-30.

[5] Dettenborn L, Tietze A, Bruckner F, Lirschbaum C. Higher cortisol content in hair among long-term unemployed individuals compared to controls. Psychoneuroendocrinology 2010;35(9):1404-9.

[6] Steptoe A, Phil D, Brydon L, Kunz-Ebrecht S. Changes in financial strain over three years, ambulatory blood pressure, and cortisol response to awakening. Psychosomatic Med 2005;67:281-7.

[7] Gundersen C, Mahatmya D, Garasky S, Lohman B. Linking psychosocial stressors and childhood obesity. Obser Rev 2011;12(5):e54-63.

[8] Chichlowska KL, Rose KM, Diez-Roux AV, et al. Life course socioeconomic conditions and metabolic syndrome in adults: the Atherosclerosis Risk in Communities (ARIC) Study. Ann Epidemiol 2009;19:875-83.

[9] Lidfeldt J, Li TY, Hu FB, Manson JE, Kawachi I. A prospective study of childhood and adult socioeconomic status and incidence of type 2 diabetes in women. Am J Epidemiol 2007;165:882-9.

[10] Galobardes B, Smith GD, Lynch JW. Systematic review of the influence of childhood socioeconomic circumstances on risk for cardiovascular disease in adulthood. Ann Epidemiol 2006;16:91-104.

[11] Careerbuilder.com. Percentage of U.S. workers living paycheck to paycheck reaches recession era low, finds careerbuilder survey[internet]. Careerbuilder.com; 2012 [cited 2013 Jul 1]. Available from: http://www.careerbuilder.com/share/aboutus/pressreleasesdetail.aspx?sd=8%2F15%2F2012&id=pr711&ed=12%2F31%2F2012.

[12] Casey T, Maldonado H. Worst off -- single-parent families in the United States: a cross-national comparison of single parenthood in the U.S. and sixteen other high-income countries [Internet]. New York; Legal Momentum; 2012 [cited 2013 Aug 26]. Available from: http://www.legalmomentum.org/sites/default/files/reports/worst-off-single-parent.pdf

[13] Nebraska Department of Health and Human Services. Smoking among Nebraska adults, 2009. Nebraska Behavioral Risk Factor Surveillance System [internet]. 2010 Jun [cited 2013 Jul 1]; Volume 1, Issue 5. Available from: http://dhhs.ne.gov/publichealth/Documents/Vol1-Issue5.pdf

[14] Nebraska Department of Health and Human Services Data. Overweight and obesity among Nebraska adults, 2010. Nebraska Behavioral Risk Surveillance System [internet]. 2011 May [cited 2013 Jul 1];

Volume 2, Issue 1. Available from: http://dhhs.ne.gov/publichealth/Documents/vol2-iss1-Overweight-obesity.pdf

[15] Nebraska Department of Health and Human Services Data. Physical activity among Nebraska adults, 2009. Nebraska Behavioral Risk Surveillance System [internet]. 2010 May (cited 2013 Jul 1]; Volume 1; Issue 2. Available from: http://dhhs.ne.gov/publichealth/Documents/Vol1-Issue2.pdf

[16] Nebraska Department of Health and Human Services Data. Behavioral Risk Factor Web Query System, 2010. Nebraska Behavioral Risk Surveillance System [internet]. 2010 [cited 2013 Jul 1]. Available from: http://public-dhhs.ne.gov/Brfss/

[17] Nebraska Department of Health and Human Services Data. Behavioral Risk Factor Web Query System, 2009. Nebraska Risk Surveillance System [internet]. 2009 [cited 2013 Jul 1]. Available from: http://public-dhhs.ne.gov/Brfss/QueryResults.aspx

[18] HealthyPeople.gov [Internet]. Washington: U.S. Department of Health and Human Services [updated 2013 Aug 28; cited 2013 Aug 30]. Heart Disease and Stroke. Available from: http://www.healthypeople.gov/2020/topicsobjectives2020/objectiveslist.aspx?topicId=21

[19] Health Functions Steering Committee. 10 essential services of public health. Public Health Functions Steering Committee, 1994.

[20] Miller WR, Rollnick S. Motivational Interviewing: Preparing People for Change 2002. Guilford Press, New York.

[21] Martins RG, Carvalho IP. Breaking bad news: Patients' preferences and health locus of control. Patient Education and Counseling 2013;92: 67-73.

[22] Sundin O, Lisspers, J, Homan-Bang C, Nygren A, Ryden L, Ohman A. Comparing multifactorial lifestyle interventions and stress management in coronary risk reduction. Int Journal of Behavioral Medicine 2003; 10(3):191-204.

[23] Bollini AM, Walker EF, Hamann S, Kestler L. The influence of perceived control and locus of control on the cortisol and subjective responses to stress. Biological Psychology 2004;67:245-260.

[24] Child and Adolescent Health Measurement Initiative. National survey of children's health, 2007 Data Resource Center [internet]. 2007 [cited 2013 Jul 1]. Available from: http://www.childhealthdata.org/docs/nsch-docs/nebraska-pdf.pdf

In: Public Health
Editors: Rosemary M. Caron and Joav Merrick

ISBN: 978-1-63321-569-6

Chapter 7

An inter-governmental approach to childhood obesity

Christine Bozlak[*1], *Adam Becker*[2,3], *Jennifer Herd*[4], *Andrew Teitelman*[5], *Judah Viola*[6], *Bradley Olson*[6] *and Bechara Choucair*[4]

[1]Department of Health Policy, Management, and Behavior, School of Public Health, University at Albany, Rensselaer, New York,
[2]Consortium to Lower Obesity in Chicago Children, Chicago, Illinois,
[3]Northwestern University, Evanston, Illinois,
[4]Chicago Department of Public Health, Chicago, Illinois,
[5]Chicago Housing Authority, Chicago, Illinois,
[6]National Louis University, Chicago, Illinois, US

Childhood obesity continues to be a global epidemic. Prevention of this public health problem requires an inter-disciplinary and social ecological approach. This chapter describes the history, function, and structure of the City of Chicago's Inter-Departmental Task Force on Childhood Obesity (IDTF), a government coalition created in 2006 by four city agencies in Chicago with the support of staff from a multi-sectoral obesity prevention coalition, to confront the rising epidemic. Now with eleven member agencies, this award-winning task force offers lessons learned for other localities working to take a governmental approach to confront one of the greatest public health threats of our time. Recommendations are provided for governments of any size to consider as they address this global public health crisis.

[*] Corresponding author: Christine Bozlak, PhD, MPH, Assistant Professor, University at Albany, School of Public Health, Department of Health Policy, Management, and Behavior, One University Place, Room 173, Rensselaer, NY 12144, United States. E-mail: cbozlak@albany.edu.

Introduction

Over the last three decades, childhood obesity (1-3) has emerged as a significant public health crisis in the United States (4) and around the world (5). Almost 35 million of the 42 million children under the age of five who are overweight are located in developing countries (6). In the United States, childhood obesity is a major concern, with researchers there predicting that this generation of American children will be the first to have a shorter lifespan than the preceding generation (4,7). Although some age groups (8) and localities, such as New York City and Los Angeles (9), are beginning to demonstrate decreases in childhood obesity rates, disparities still exist; especially for children in lower-income, African American, and Latino communities (10).

According to data analyzed by the Consortium to Lower Obesity in Chicago Children (CLOCC), in Chicago, Illinois, young children in this city have had considerably higher obesity rates than children in the rest of Illinois and across the US. However, there are signs of improvement. Data analyzed by CLOCC show a decrease in obesity prevalence among 3-7 year olds over a five year period. A recent report indicates declines in obesity exclusively among Chicago Public School students (11). These improvements cannot be attributed to one intervention but are, in part, the result of significant coordination of obesity efforts in Chicago since 2002 (3). One important aspect of this coordination is the City of Chicago's Inter-Departmental Task Force on Childhood Obesity (IDTF). The purpose of this work is to align and coordinate Chicago governmental agency efforts to plan, implement, and evaluate policy, systems, and environmental change (PSE) strategies to address the childhood obesity epidemic in Chicago. The task force prioritizes children between the ages of 0-18. However, the IDTF acknowledges that early intervention is critical and thus interventions tailored for the early childhood years of 0-5 are emphasized.

Background of government collaboration on childhood obesity prevention

Public health experts widely acknowledge that government has an essential role to play in protecting the public's health (12,13). In the United States, state and local governments are authorized to protect the public's health, a concept known as "police power," and there is well-established precedent for government to exercise this power for childhood obesity prevention. For example, state and local governments have exercised this power to require the posting of nutritional information in restaurants, regulate the sale of junk food in schools, and impose zoning restrictions to limit the location of fast food establishments (14). Government is in a unique position to assess public health problems and coordinate implementation of policies, programs, and services to alleviate these issues (1,13). Additionally, public health experts recognize the importance of an interdisciplinary approach with non-health governmental agencies' participation in the protection of the public's health (1).

Through Internet research and discussions with health departments across the US, the authors found that other obesity-focused government coalitions and task forces, such as those in the cities of New York, Boston, Baltimore, and Columbus, tend to convene for a delimited time to develop an agenda and work on specific topics on an as-needed basis. Some are created formally by legislation and others are developed based upon a call from a local government entity. Although other childhood obesity prevention task forces may exist, the authors believe that the City of Chicago's Inter-Departmental Task Force on Childhood Obesity is unique given the length of time it has been operational, its multi-pronged and multi-sector approach, and the city's ongoing commitment to its existence.

Background of Chicago's intergovernmental approach to childhood obesity prevention

The City of Chicago, situated in Northern Illinois, with a population of over 2.7 million (15) is a diverse urban area governed by a Mayor and City Council. In 2002, forty childhood obesity advocates convened to discuss a coordinated approach to the childhood obesity epidemic in Chicago (3,16). This discussion resulted in the establishment of the Consortium to Lower Obesity in Chicago Children (CLOCC), housed at Ann and Robert H. Lurie Children's Hospital of Chicago. This network connects hundreds of organizations to support, coordinate, and unite partners to promote healthy and active lifestyles for children and families. Consortium partners use data to guide their efforts and frame their priorities. For example, prevalence data collected from student health records and community-based surveys have helped to prioritize age groups and geographic locations within the City for intervention. Environmental audit data collected by researchers and community members (e.g., street and sidewalk conditions, merchandise in food retail establishments) have helped partners to prioritize strategies to improve access to healthy food and safe opportunities for physical activity. CLOCC's primary focus is on children aged zero to five, their caregivers, and their communities. CLOCC's work cuts across medical, government, corporate, academic, advocacy, and other sectors. Currently, more than 3,000 individuals representing over 1,300 organizations participate in the Consortium.

CLOCC initially engaged the government sector by creating a Governmental Policies and Programs working group. Co-chaired by representatives from two city agencies, the Chicago Department of Public Health and the Chicago Department of Family and Support Services, this working group was comprised of representatives from government agencies (including those who participated in the IDTF) and non-governmental organizations interested in policy (e.g., social service organizations, advocacy organizations dedicated to the prevention of obesity-related diseases, legal organizations that prioritize child health issues). Over time, CLOCC and city government leadership recognized the need for inter-governmental collaboration separate from efforts that included non-governmental partners.

In 2006, CLOCC's leadership approached the Chicago Department of Public Health (CDPH) with the idea of creating the Inter-Departmental Task Force on Childhood Obesity (IDTF). As the lead government agency, CDPH invited the Chicago Public Schools (CPS), the Chicago Department of Family and Support Services (DFSS), and the Chicago Park District (Parks) to join the effort. Since that time, seven other city agencies have joined (Table 1). In 2007, the IDTF hosted an event in a national series of "town-hall" meetings to gather input about childhood obesity. Six hundred Chicagoans attended the event, demonstrated support for the emerging IDTF, and helped develop its priorities.

Our project

The IDTF was created to develop a coordinated governmental response to the childhood obesity epidemic in Chicago. This multi-agency approach was based on the premise that the complexity of childhood obesity requires inter-disciplinary solutions. City governments, because they are comprised of a range of agencies with diverse expertise, have an important opportunity to coordinate across disciplines (1). In 2006, the founding four IDTF agencies established the mission: "Chicago's city government will play a leading role in confronting childhood obesity through an unprecedented level of coordination, the strategic provision of services, and the advancement of evidence-based practices and policies to improve nutrition and physical activity in a wellness-enhancing environment." The IDTF follows a social ecological approach to childhood obesity prevention, meaning that its interventions are focused on the environments in which children are developing (2); not solely on the children themselves.

To accomplish its mission, the IDTF meets monthly. Each department's leader designates one or more staff members to represent their agency; most often those whose day-to-day work aligns most closely with IDTF objectives. The Commissioner of Health periodically convenes an IDTF leadership meeting to update the other agency executives on progress and future plans. Each year, the IDTF sets annual objectives, using a three-pronged strategic approach as a guiding framework.

Strategy #1: Primary Prevention

The Task Force's primary prevention activities are intended to reach all children in Chicago. These activities include public education, data surveillance, environmental assessments, coordinated policymaking, and professional development for agency staff. The IDTF adopted CLOCC's 5-4-3-2-1 Go!® healthy lifestyle message which provides daily recommendations for children and families related to nutrition, physical activity, and screen-time (see www.clocc.net/partners/54321Go). Since 2008, the Task Force has disseminated 5-4-3-2-1 Go!® by distributing materials throughout city facilities. In 2009, the IDTF contributed to a city-wide campaign to disseminate the message to 1.5 million Chicagoans with 8 million media impressions. Evaluation of the campaign suggests that those exposed to the message were more likely to adopt certain healthy behaviors than those who were not exposed (17).

A number of trainings delivered by IDTF member agencies were opened to staff from other IDTF agencies. The Department of Family and Support Services (DFSS) has invited partners to trainings on nutrition and physical activity in early childhood settings. The Park District has invited partners to physical activity trainings. These cross-training opportunities help to expand the capacity of city staff members who interact with young children.

In terms of surveillance, the Chicago Department of Public Health and Chicago Public Schools have a five-year inter-governmental agreement to share de-identified student health data collected through required health examinations at school entry, sixth grade, and ninth grade. CLOCC provided technical assistance on analysis methods that mirrored those implemented by the U.S. Centers for Disease Control and Prevention (CDC). The City published the first report on obesity prevalence among CPS students, which has helped guide the IDTF and the public health community to the areas in the city with the highest rates (11). A second report was released in late 2013 and showed a slight decline in childhood obesity rates among CPS kindergarten-aged students (18).

Table 1. Inter-Departmental Task Force on Childhood Obesity Membership

IDTF Member Agency Name	Associated Acronym
Chicago Department of Public Health (lead agency)	CDPH
Chicago Department of Family and Support Services	DFSS
Chicago Department of Planning and Development	DPD
Chicago Department of Transportation	CDOT
Chicago Housing Authority	CHA
Chicago Park District	Parks
Chicago Police Department	CPD
Chicago Public Library	CPL
Chicago Public Schools	CPS
Chicago Transit Authority	CTA
Mayor's Office for People with Disabilities	MOPD
*Technical assistance provided by the Consortium to Lower Obesity in Chicago Children	CLOCC

Strategy #2: Early childhood

The Task Force prioritizes activities that are focused on enhancing early childhood environments. Evidence increasingly points to the need to intervene early in order to curb the childhood obesity epidemic (19). In the US, infants and young children are increasingly cared for outside their home (20), thus, early childhood settings are a key context for childhood obesity intervention (21). As of 2011, there were almost 84,000 slots in licensed child care centers and homes in Chicago, demonstrating the potential reach of interventions when implemented in Chicago child care settings (22).

The IDTF's primary approach to early childhood is to strengthen the practices of childcare providers under the purview of city agencies. CDPH and DFSS led a policy change initiative to ensure that standards for nutrition, physical activity, and screen time in Chicago licensed childcare settings under CDPH's jurisdiction aligned with best practices. In 2009, CDPH and the Chicago Board of Health passed a joint resolution to this effect (23). CDPH then partnered with CLOCC and two other local non-profit organizations to provide training to childcare providers to support implementation of the standards.

Strategy #3: Geographic hubs

IDTF members developed a strategy that focuses on aligning partner resources in key geographic areas of Chicago where childhood obesity rates are expected or known to be highest. Known as Wellness Campuses, these areas of geographic concentration helped agencies to focus on priority neighborhoods and to align efforts for educational, programmatic, and clinical childhood obesity prevention services for children and their families. Early wellness campuses were anchored by Chicago Park District "Wellness Centers" – park district facilities equipped to provide enhanced fitness programming for youth. A 2009 CLOCC study found that when more resources and staff training were devoted to youth fitness through the Wellness Center structure, children engaged in more intensive physical activity for a longer period of time than those in parks without the centers. Other IDTF partners directed their activities to these geographic areas. For example, the Chicago Department of Transportation's (CDOT) Bike Ambassadors provide bicycle safety education at Wellness Centers.

Chicago Public Schools and the Chicago Park District identified ways to collaborate so that students in schools, including early childhood settings, with limited facilities for physical activity can use park resources. For example, through the Healthy Chicago Public Schools initiative, forty park sites have included thirty minutes of structured physical activity time in their existing early childhood programs. In addition, Chicago Park District staff members have been trained in the SPARK (www.sparkpe.org) early childhood program to promote physical activity in this population. The next step will be to connect nearby CPS schools who offer pre-kindergarten to the parks where the SPARK physical activity program will be implemented. The Chicago Park District staff trained in SPARK can also provide the training to CPS teachers.

More recently, other departmental strategies are anchoring geographically-defined settings around the city, and IDTF members are exploring opportunities to align their resources in these emerging locations. For example, CDOT is establishing "safety zones" where a variety of traffic-calming and enforcement approaches will be concentrated around schools and parks. CPS recently received funding from a U.S. Centers for Disease Control and Prevention's Community Transformation Grant to create "healthy school zones" that combine school wellness activities with efforts to improve the external food and activity environments. By focusing these collaborative efforts in the same geographic locations, the city has a coordinated approach in neighborhoods where obesity is a significant problem.

Findings

In addition to providing a foundation for collaborative alignment of existing resources, IDTF members have been able to leverage single opportunities into larger initiatives. The IDTF has been a foundation for new funding; expanding the capacity of city agencies to intervene to address childhood obesity in Chicago. In 2010, Chicago embarked on its largest federally-funded obesity prevention project to date, Healthy Places. This $5.8 million project was funded through a cooperative agreement from the Centers for Disease Control and Prevention (CDC) between CLOCC and the CDC under the U.S. Department of Health and Human Services' Communities Putting Prevention to Work initiative (CPPW). CLOCC served as the bona fide agent for the City of Chicago and led the effort in partnership with CDPH. The overall goal of Healthy Places was to implement sustainable policy, systems, and environmental changes that address obesity in Chicago by creating healthier environments where Chicagoans live, work, learn, and play. Several of the project's outcome objectives were integrated into "Healthy Chicago," the City of Chicago's official public health agenda (24).

Through the Healthy Places initiative, IDTF agencies worked together on projects, such as design guidelines for "complete streets," a framework that supports multi-modal use of streets with an emphasis on pedestrian and cyclist safety; a healthy food plan to guide government action to address access to healthy foods, and a safe park access plan, called "Make Way for Play." Although the federal funding period has ended, IDTF members are establishing mechanisms for ensuring the sustainability of Healthy Places efforts.

Evaluation of the IDTF

The Institute of Medicine (1) stresses the need to evaluate local obesity prevention efforts and encourage partnerships with local universities in this effort. In 2011, the IDTF commissioned an evaluation of its work and hired, with funding from CLOCC, two external researchers from a local university to work collaboratively with the Task Force to identify successes, challenges, and opportunities for improvement.

The evaluation identified outcomes in three main areas: 1) policy, 2) education, and 3) programs. Evaluation data pointed to a number of policy outcomes resulting from IDTF collaborations. The implementation of improved childcare standards, as well as policies for healthy vending across several member agencies, were found to be important policy outcomes. Programmatic outcomes included Safe Routes to School implementation, Open Streets (a day-long event that closes streets to vehicular traffic and opens them for recreational use), the Park District's fitness-related training, the dissemination of 5-4-3-2-1 Go!®, and the Healthy Places initiatives. The evaluation also found that the IDTF wellness campus initiative is a comprehensive concept in that it covers both physical activity and healthy eating promotion within the various community settings in which children interact.

IDTF members continue to integrate lessons learned from the evaluation into process improvements and intervention design. Evaluation results were shared with CDPH after transition to a new commissioner to keep the Department invested in the IDTF. In 2013, the IDTF began to explore options for an evaluation of the health impacts of the IDTF on Chicago children.

Discussion

Establishing a coordinated, local governmental response to childhood obesity prevention is a critical strategy to address this epidemic (1). The experiences of the IDTF in Chicago can be helpful to other communities considering a similar, government-led, multi-disciplinary effort. The following recommendations are provided by IDTF members based on the IDTF evaluation findings.

1. Strong leadership: Identify one partner to lead with one or more dedicated staff members to coordinate the effort. Leadership from a government entity, ideally the health department, can help to keep city leadership informed and can provide access

to city resources. In Chicago, CLOCC's expertise on childhood obesity enabled them to add technical and content support to CDPH's leadership. Communities with similar non-governmental entities might consider their inclusion to provide similar support. On a regular basis, it is helpful for the task force to obtain an official endorsement of its work from local governmental leaders. With the IDTF, this is accomplished through an annual agency leadership meeting to keep high-level decision-makers informed. This meeting also provides the leadership a platform to discuss childhood obesity issues from their vantage point.

In Chicago, there is leadership from the top. Mayor Rahm Emanuel has made focusing on the child one of his main priorities of his administration for the past two years. In addition, the City's public health agenda, "Healthy Chicago" includes obesity as one of 12 priorities and articulates the critical role of public-private partnerships in meeting the goals set forth in the agenda. This top-level support is essential for the continuation of the IDTF and the engagement of its member agencies.

2. Task force membership: Think broadly and recruit diverse agencies. It will take every sector, even those not traditionally considered as health-focused (e.g., transportation, public safety, planning and land use) working together to address this complex epidemic. It is helpful to have budgetary support for this work across agencies. Inter-agency agreements may facilitate collaboration, solidify commitments, and ensure role clarity.

   The IDTF operates under a multi-disciplinary model with mixed committee assignments to ensure that the City's member agencies, with differing missions and priorities, remain engaged in the process. IDTF member agencies also benefit from their participation in the IDTF because they know they can utilize the IDTF to leverage and support their own agency's objectives – a point emphasized in the next recommendation.
3. Maximize opportunities for collaboration: Maximize the potential for "synergy" with other efforts throughout the locality. Aligning objectives and activities with existing governmental priorities can increase the likelihood of successful implementation. Identifying ways that the collaborative work can support the individual priorities of member agencies helps to secure broad support. The work of a task force such as the IDTF could be integrated with other initiatives related to economic development, education, and public safety to accomplish other government goals.
4. Ensure effective communication: Government agency staffs are often pulled in multiple directions as leadership responds to well-established priorities and a constant stream of external pressures and demands. Organized and frequent communication among task force members can ensure that momentum is not lost even if members cannot attend every meeting. A centralized and cross-agency event calendar can help to increase awareness of member agency initiatives related to the task force and to identify opportunities for collaboration. Task force agencies can also help disseminate materials related to a partner agency's event. In addition, regularly update the local governmental leaders of the task force's work to increase support and buy-in from decision-makers. Establishing mechanisms to disseminate the task force's work and messaging to the local community and other public health

professionals is also essential to increase support and participation from these entities.

Throughout the years, the IDTF has utilized various communication mechanisms and meeting schedules. The IDTF has functioned most efficiently when there was one staff-person dedicated to communicating with all the representatives of the member agencies via email and conference calls for scheduling and project coordination purposes. It is most effective to have one individual responsible for coordinating task force communication because this person can synthesize the communication within the task force and appropriately triage and follow-up on project-related responsibilities and other task force-related items. Throughout the existence of the IDTF, monthly in-person meetings helped to advance IDTF progress on its initiatives, and they also enabled the representatives from the member agencies to establish effective working relationships that would have otherwise not developed. Over time, this resulted in an unforeseen positive outcome from the IDTF in that there has been increased communication between member agencies on non-task force-related initiatives pertaining to the well-being of Chicago residents.

Staff turnover can be a challenge for any type of coalition. For the IDTF, individual representatives from the member agencies become internal champions for the work and are critical points of contact between task force staff and each participating agency. Encouraging members to identify more than one representative can help to ensure that the IDTF remains a priority for each of its member agencies and can help prevent disruptions in communications that might occur if a member's sole representative left his or her organization.

5. Prioritize task force projects: Utilize intervention research evidence and best practice guidelines to prioritize task force projects. It may be most efficient to charge one task force member or committee with the responsibility of staying current with the latest research on effective approaches to childhood obesity prevention and communicating this information to the group. In addition, the resources of a government task force may be used most effectively when directed towards agency practices and city policy, as opposed to programs delivered to citizens, because governments are uniquely situated to focus on the former. Such policy should include modifying the environment to make healthy choices practical and available to all community members. This approach is known as "Policy, Systems, and Environmental Change" (PSE), and is increasingly utilized by U.S. public health practitioners working in chronic disease prevention. By changing laws and shaping the landscape around us, a significant and sustainable impact can be made, often with fewer resources than one-time programmatic interventions with limited reach.

In addition to these recommendations, the challenges of creating and sustaining a task force of this nature must be recognized. It can be extremely helpful to measure the successes and challenges of the task force. Evidence of progress can help to keep city leaders engaged and identification of challenges can help the members to overcome them or prevent them in the future. Childhood obesity, because it is a chronic condition, may not be prioritized by governmental leadership amidst other, perhaps more visible issues (e.g., crime, academic achievement). Using data to illustrate the connections between childhood obesity and other priority health and/or social problems can help garner and maintain support. Finally, the current fiscal and structural challenges experienced by many local governments in the U.S., such as staff turnover, hiring freezes, and resource shortages, must also be considered when prioritizing work for the task force.

The City of Chicago's Inter-Departmental Task Force on Childhood Obesity is a unique entity that, since 2006, has grown to include eleven city agencies collaborating to effectively plan and implement childhood obesity prevention strategies. The work involves a broad cross-section of the governmental sector, including transit, housing, education, parks, health, urban planning, libraries, and public safety.

Since its creation, the IDTF has received national recognition for its innovative work. The IDTF strategy has also been presented at national conferences. In 2011, the Chicago Department of Public Health received a Model Practice Award from the National Association of County and City Health Officials for the IDTF. Most recently, the City of Chicago was recognized for its multi-sector obesity prevention efforts by the National League of Cities for its achievement in the Let's Move! Cities, Towns and Counties program. The City received this award in large part because of the accomplishments made possible by the IDTF collectively and its individual members.

Chicago's Inter-Departmental Task Force on Childhood Obesity illustrates the critical function of government agencies in tackling a complex public health problem. While not solely responsible for them, the IDTF has contributed to the steady declines in childhood obesity prevalence described earlier. Research evidence and national experts support the premise that the kinds of policy and environmental changes brought about by the IDTF do lead to improved nutritional and physical activity behaviors in children, which in turn result in improvements in population-level obesity rates. The experience of the IDTF can serve as a model for government leadership at the local level and demonstrates the important role that every government sector can and should play in reducing this epidemic among its most vulnerable and youngest citizens.

Acknowledgments

The authors wish to thank the Otho SA Sprague Memorial Institute, the Michael and Susan Dell Foundation, and the Robert Wood Johnson Foundation for funding CLOCC's staff support of the IDTF, Dr. Matt Longjohn for his advocacy that helped create the Task Force, and all the IDTF agencies and agency representatives who contributed to this work since 2006.

References

[1] Institute of Medicine. Local government actions to prevent childhood obesity. Washington, DC: National Academies Press, 2009.

[2] Davison K, Birch, L. Childhood overweight: a contextual model and recommendations for future research. Obes Rev 2001;2(3):159-71.

[3] Becker A, Longjohn M, Christoffel K. Taking on childhood obesity in a big city: Consortium to Lower Obesity in Chicago Children (CLOCC). Prog Pediatr Cardiol 2008;25(2):199-206.

[4] US Department of Health and Human Services. The Surgeon General's call to action to prevent and decrease overweight and obesity. Washington, DC: US Government Printing Office, 2001.

[5] Prentice, A. The emerging epidemic of obesity in developing countries. Int J Epidemiol 2006;35(1):93-9.

[6] deOnis M, Blössner M, Borghi E. Global prevalence and trends of overweight and obesity among preschool children. Am J Clin Nutr 2010;92(5):1257-64.

[7] Olshansky J, Passaro D, Hershow R, Layden J, Carnes B, Brody J, et al. A potential decline in life expectancy in the United States in the 21st century. N Engl J Med 2005;352(11):1138-45.

[8] Ogden C, Carroll M, Curtin L, Lamb M, Flegal K. Prevalence of high body mass index in US children and adolescents, 2007-2008. JAMA 2010;303(3):242-49.

[9] US Department of Health and Human Services Centers for Disease Control and Prevention. Obesity prevalence among low income, preschool-aged children – New York City and Los Angeles County, 2003-2011. MMWR 2013;62(2).

[10] Trust for America's Health. F as in Fat: How obesity threatens America's future 2012. 2013. Accessed 2012 November 20. URL: http://healthyamericans.org/report/100/

[11] City of Chicago. Overweight and obesity among Chicago public schools students, 2010-2011. 2013. Accessed 20 November 2013. URL: http://www.cityofchicago.org/content/dam/city/depts/cdph/CDPH/Over weightObesityReportFeb272013.pdf

[12] Jochelson K. Nanny or steward? The role of government in public health. Public Health 2006;120(12):1149-55.

[13] Turnock BJ. Public health: what it is and how it works, 4th ed. Burlington, MA: Jones and Bartlett, 2009.

[14] Mermin SE, Graff SK. A legal primer for the obesity prevention movement. Am J Health Behav 2009;99(10):1799-05.

[15] U.S. Census Bureau. State & County Quickfacts: Chicago, IL 2010. Accessed 2013 November 1. URL: http://quickfacts.census.gov/qfd/states/17/1714000.html

[16] Longjohn MM. Chicago project uses ecological approach to obesity prevention. Pediatr Ann 2004;33(1):55-7.

[17] Evans WD, Christoffel KK, Necheles K, Becker AB, Snider J. Outcomes of the 5-4-3-2-1 Go! childhood obesity community trial. Am J Health Behav 2011;35(2):189-98.

[18] City of Chicago. Healthy Chicago spotlight childhood obesity. Chicago, Illinois: City of Chicago, 2013. Accessed 20 November 2013. URL: http://www.cityofchicago.org/content/dam/city/depts/cdph/CDPH/HCO besityReport10302013.pdf

[19] Nader P, Huang T, Gahagan S, Kumanyika S, Hammond R, Christoffel K. Next steps in obesity prevention: Altering early life system to support healthy parents, infants, and toddlers. Child Obes 2012;8(3):195-204.

[20] Baker M, Gruber J, Milligan K. Universal child care, maternal labor supply, and family well-being. J Polit Econ 2008;116(4):709-45.

[21] Kaphingst K, Story M. Child care as an untapped setting for obesity prevention: state child care licensing regulations related to nutrition, physical activity, and media use for preschool-aged children in the United States. Prev Chronic Dis 2009;6(1):A11.

[22] Illinois Action for Children Research Department. Child care providers and capacity by Cook County Municipality. 2013. Accessed 2013 November 1. URL: http://www.actforchildren.org/site/DocServer/Commonly_Requested_C hild_Care_Data_by_Cook_Municipality_.pdf?docID=2123

[23] Bozlak C, Becker A. Using Evidence to Create Active Communities: Stories from the Field—Policy and Research with Chicago's Child Care Centers: a Commentary to Accompany the Active Living Research Supplement to Annals of Behavioral Medicine. Ann Behav Med 2013;45Suppl 1:s11-s13.

[24] Chicago Department of Public Health. Healthy Chicago Agenda. 2013. Accessed 2013 November 1. URL: http://www.cityofchicago.org/city/en/depts/cdph/provdrs/healthychicago.html

In: Public Health
Editors: Rosemary M. Caron and Joav Merrick

ISBN: 978-1-63321-569-6

Chapter 8

Peer teen advocates and increased awareness of human papillomavirus and vaccination among urban youth

***Denise Uyar*[1*], *Staci Young*[2], *Sarah Tyree-Francis*[3] *and Mary Ann Kiepczynski*[4]**

[1]Medical College of Wisconsin Department of Obstetrics and Gynecology, Division of Gynecology Oncology,
[2]Medical College of Wisconsin, Department of Family and Community Medicine,
[3]Adolescent Holistic Health Initiatives, Don and Sallie Davis Boys and Girls Club and
[4]City of Milwaukee Health Department, Disease Control & Environmental Health, Public Health Nurse Immunization Program Coordinator, Milwaukee, Wisconsin, US

The city of Milwaukee, Wisconsin ranks among the highest urban areas for sexually transmitted disease in the United States with human papillomavirus being one of the most common sexually transmitted infections. In 2006, the Advisory Committee on Immunization Practices recommended routine vaccination of adolescent girls at ages 11 or 12 years with 3 doses of the Food and Drug Administration approved HPV vaccination. Despite the availability, safety and demonstrated efficacy of these vaccines, only 33% of adolescent girls in the United States have received all three doses of the series. In Milwaukee, less than 30% of adolescents have received the vaccination series. Several studies have evaluated the barriers for HPV vaccination. Consistently, deficits in knowledge and education for both parents and adolescents regarding HPV and the vaccination are cited as reasons why youth did not get the vaccine. This study was created to determine if today's urban youth could successfully be engaged in a program of positive health messaging surrounding HPV and the HPV vaccination using peer educators and social media.

* Corresponding author: Denise Uyar, MD Medical College of Wisconsin, Associate Professor Department of Obstetrics and Gynecology, Division of Gynecology Oncology 9200 West Wisconsin Avenue, Milwaukee, WI 53226, United States. E-mail: duyar@mcw.edu.

Introduction

Human papillomavirus (HPV) infection is the most common sexually transmitted infection in the United States (1). Approximately 79 million persons in the United States are infected with HPV and approximately 14 million will become infected each year (2). HPV is not a reported infection, but its rates are believed to mirror that of other reportable infections, such as chlamydia and gonorrhea. Prevalence rates have been documented based on seroprevalence (3-5). Human papillomaviruses (HPVs) are typically acquired within the first months of sexual initiation. The peak incidence occurs among men and women ages 15-24 years (4). Persistent HPV infection is associated with a spectrum of health concerns from condyloma and anogenital pre-cancers to cervical, vulvar, vaginal, anal, penile and some oropharyngeal malignancies (6). Cervical cancer has been entirely attributed to persistent HPV infection with high risk viral types (HPV 16 and HPV 18) (7). In the United States, approximately 11,000 cases of cervical cancer are diagnosed each year with 4,000 women dying of the disease annually despite effective screening for cervical cancer (8). The direct cost of treatment of HPV-related diseases is approximately $4 billion per year in the United States. The vaccination is not intended to replace cervical cancer screening, but combined with increased compliance with screening measures it represents a potential cost-effective dual strategy ultimately resulting in decreased HPV morbidity and mortality (9,10). HPV infections and their associated morbidity have been found to disproportionately affect racial and ethnic minority populations in the United States (11,12). Thus, specific subgroups of youth are at particularly high risk. Nearly one quarter of 14-19 year olds are infected with HPV but the greatest prevalence is noted among low-income minorities (13). Lack of uptake of the HPV vaccination of this subgroup has raised concerns that the current disparity seen in HPV infection morbidity and mortality will grow ever wider in the future (14). HPV infection, therefore, represents a significant health concern for all, but especially for vulnerable minority youths where rates of sexually transmitted diseases are known to be highest (15). Two prophylactic HPV vaccines are available and have been approved by the Food and Drug Administration (FDA). The Advisory Committee on Immunization Practices (ACIP) recommends vaccination for both males and females for ages 11-12 years with catch up vaccination from age 13 until age 26 years. Both the quadrivalent and bivalent vaccines protect against infection with high risk HPV 16 and HPV 18 which cause 70% of cervical cancers and the majority of other HPV-associated cancers. The quadrivalent vaccination also protects against low risk HPV 6 and HPV 11 which cause 90% of genital warts (16,17). The efficacy and safety of the vaccination has been established with long term evaluation (16,18,19). Clinical trials have established 90-100% efficacy for the prevention of precancerous cervical lesions for these vaccines when given prior to initiation of sexual activity (18,20). The potential public health impact of these vaccinations has not been realized as it depends largely on vaccination acceptability and uptake among the target youth population and especially among groups disproportionately affected by HPV within the population.

In the United States, the 2007-2012 National Immunization Survey-Teen (NIS-Teen) reported that only 54% of girls have received one or more doses of the HPV series and only 33% have received all 3 doses to complete the HPV series (2). HPV vaccination rates have unfortunately stalled in the United States with no observed increase in vaccination rates from

2011 to 2012 (2). The barriers to HPV vaccination acceptance and uptake are multifactorial and include factors such as parental acceptability of HPV vaccination, adolescent acceptability of the HPV vaccination, physician acceptability of vaccination and endorsement, and vaccine access (21,22). Frequently, lack of knowledge, on the part of parents, adolescents and physicians, is a central theme surrounding lack of vaccination (23). Several studies have pointed out the need for more tailored approaches to increasing vaccination acceptability (14,24).

Although there has been almost universal agreement that HPV infection is an increasing health burden, particularly affecting minority youth and that a new strategy for increasing vaccination rates is needed, there seemed to be very few strategies proposed to start addressing the current deficits. This project proposes a tailored approach to specifically address deficits in HPV and HPV vaccination knowledge among urban minority youth in Milwaukee, Wisconsin. The HPV vaccination rate in Milwaukee is less than 30% (personal communication city of Milwaukee Health Department), far below the national average and the established targets for Healthy People 2020 (25), demonstrating a large need for increased HPV knowledge and awareness in our community. A partnership led by the Medical College of Wisconsin (MCW), the Boys & Girls Clubs of Greater Milwaukee (BGCGM) and the City of Milwaukee Health Department (MHD) utilized peer teen educators and social media to achieve project objectives. Partners received funding from MCW's Healthier Wisconsin Partnership Program.

Our study

The MCW Institutional Review Board (IRB) approval was obtained prior to recruiting or consenting participants.

Recruitment and training. Youth were eligible to participate in the program if they were between 13-19 years of age. Participants were recruited from the BGCGM, a national non-profit organization that provides after school services to urban youth; Milwaukee has program sites throughout the city. BGCGM is the oldest and largest youth serving agency in the city with 38 locations. All participants received stipends for their participation at specified levels of the project to ensure that participants completed the program. Six youth age 15 and over were recruited as team leaders for this study. Team leaders received $10 for each team member recruited and $25 for completing the extra 60 -90 minute training session. Participants that completed the pre and post-tests received $25. Each participant received $25 for completion of the storyboard or preliminary design of the project. Each team member received $100 for completion of the project in its entirety. Attendance at the 2nd Annual PSA Premiere held in downtown Milwaukee was awarded $25. The winning team members of the individual campaigns in each category (PSA, billboard or brochure) were awarded $50.

Leaders participated in an age appropriate HPV informational session created by MCW and MHD about the HPV virus, sexually transmitted disease and protection from infection which included discussions about vaccination, condom use and abstinence. These team leaders then recruited up to five team members from BGCGM or associated programs for their group. A total of 30 team members were enrolled in this study. Study participants were both male and female. The six team leaders were responsible for organizing their group and arranging the HPV training session for their group. All participants completed pre- and post-training surveys to assess their HPV knowledge (see figure 1).

Educational intervention. After the training sessions, youth participants discussed and decided their choice of media for presentation: public service announcements (PSA), brochures or city billboards. Brainstorming sessions were also performed concurrently among team members and study coordinators to discuss a "brand" for the HPV project including a logo and website. Participants completed a survey to identify their preferred social media platforms; Twitter and Facebook were the most preferred methods of communication. Participants received education on responsible social media use and signed a contract to ensure that they utilized it responsibly. Teams used Twitter, Instagram, and Facebook to coordinate their meetings and to inform their peers about the program.

Groups were assigned to one of their first two choices of media for presentation and paired with a volunteer community mentor with media expertise. Two groups created individual finished products in each category; at the completion of the program there were two PSA videos, two billboards campaigns and two brochures. Groups met at least bi-weekly for four months with mentors to create and formalize their ideas in their respective categories. Partners purchased the domain name *itsjust3hpv.org* and developed into an interactive website including a logo created by the youth (Fig 2.). Website functionality enabled our study team to track votes the first two weeks and visits on a monthly basis. All of the completed products displayed the website and logo for heightened community awareness and project visibility.

Post and Retrospective Pretest Measures

DATE: ________ **GENDER (Circle one):** Female Male Transgender **AGE:** ________

RACE/ETHNICITY (Circle one): Black/African American White/Caucasian Latino/Hispanic Native American

Asian American Other: ________ **ZIP CODE:** ________

Instructions: Look at learning areas #1-8. Tell us what you knew *before* you started this program <u>AND</u> what you know *after* participating in this program.

BEFORE participating in this program... **AFTER participating in this program...**

Was Poor	Was Fair	Was Good	Was Excellent	**Learning Areas**	Is Poor	Is Fair	Is Good	Is Excellent
				1.My awareness of HPV.				
				2.My knowledge of HPV.				
				3.My understanding of the risk factors for contracting HPV.				
				4.My knowledge of the health risks associated with HPV.				
				5.My knowledge of how to protect myself against HPV.				
				6.My awareness of the need for the HPV vaccine for females.				
				7.My awareness of the need for HPV vaccine for males.				
				8. My understanding of where to get the HPV vaccine for free.				

Figure 1. Pre- and post-training survey.

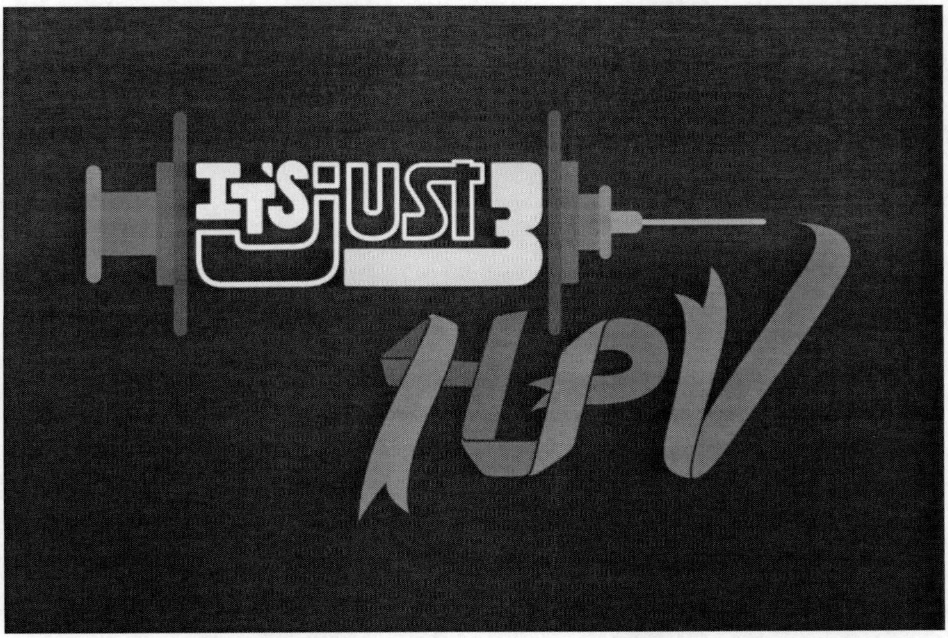

Figure 2. HPV project logo created by project participants.

Findings

A total 28 youth (94%) completed this project; 23 participants (83%) were female and 5 participants (17%) were male. Ages of participants ranged from 14-18 and they all resided in the city of Milwaukee. Participants identified themselves as African American, Latino or Native American, with only one identified as "other, not otherwise specified" and one who did not designate ethnicity.

The survey results indicated that 83% of participants completed the pre- and post-training surveys (see figure 1). The pre-training surveys indicated primarily "poor, fair or good" responses to HPV knowledge questions with only six respondents indicating "excellent" to two or more survey questions. In contrast, on the post-survey questionnaire respondents indicated universally "good to excellent" responses to the HPV knowledge questions with only two surveys with one answer in the "poor" category.

Votes for the best project in PSAs, billboards and brochures were tracked online for a two week period and additionally with live texting at the 2nd Annual PSA Premiere, a citywide event in Milwaukee with approximately 250 youth in attendance. 557 votes were counted to determine winners in each category and the winning projects were announced and posted on the *itsjust3hpv.org* website. The unique brochure created was a tri-fold with the appearance of a cell phone which was particularly well received. The billboard exemplified the youths appeal for short messages with a striking visual. The brochure and billboard winners are shown in Figures 3 and 4. The PSA video winner is not visible in this article; videos are posted on YouTube and have been viewed over 300 times.

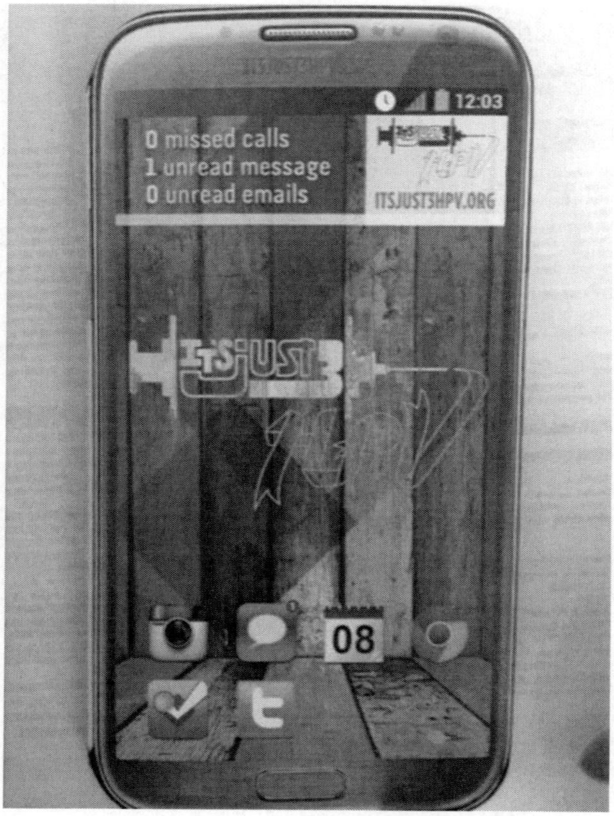

Figure 3. Winner of the HPV brochure campaign.

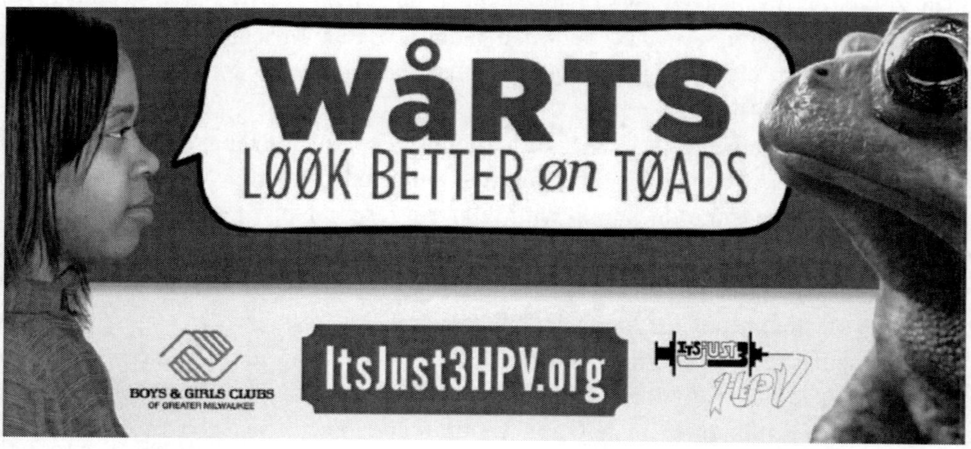
WåRTS
LØØK BETTER øn TØADS
BOYS & GIRLS CLUBS
OF GREATER MILWAUKEE
ItsJust3HPV.org

Figure 4. Winner of HPV billboard campaign.

The website includes information about HPV and HPV vaccination, links or visual images of all completed projects, and the teams of youth involved and their community mentors. Between the April 2013 launch of the website and December of 2013 there have been over 4500 visits and the website metrics reveal that it is viewed on average 35 times per day.

The winning brochure was featured on the website with an option to order copies. Partners track brochure distribution by the recipients' postal address and a questionnaire that recipients complete that includes their organization description. To date, approximately 22 individuals representing various programs requested brochures. The majority of requests are from the greater Milwaukee area but, due to the dissemination of the work at local and regional conferences, requests have come from rural Wisconsin, Minneapolis, MN, Louisville, KY and Memphis, TN. The majority of recipients identify themselves as non-for profit organizations (33%), schools (28%), community organizations (19%), or hospital or clinics (19%). The audience for their distribution is indicated as youths ages 9-20, males and females and of black, white, Latino/ Hispanic or multiracial ethnicities. Over half of the recipients (58%) indicate knowledge of the project from the website, social media or a colleague.

Discussion

The concept of this study arose from the partnership's shared goal of improved reproductive health, specifically the great need to address the low HPV vaccination rate in a city where the rates of sexually transmitted diseases are among the highest in the nation. The urban community we serve is comprised predominantly of ethnic and racial minorities as evidenced by the demographics of the youth participating in this project. The literature to date reveals many barriers to HPV vaccination but few recommendations on how to approach these issues. Fernandez et al. organized potential HPV interventions into three categories: community education, provider education and improving vaccine access (24). Our study sought to address one component of this triad: community education; specifically in adolescents, utilizing peer teen educators. Fernandez et al. noted that personal perceptions of HPV risk, personal perceptions of HPV severity, perceptions of one's peers and social norms are significant factors influencing willingness to have oneself vaccinated (24). Peer perceptions have significant influence.

Several studies have demonstrated that peer education can make a significant difference among youths. Peer educators are motivated young individuals that have undergone informal education with their peers with the intent of augmenting their own knowledge and skills to enable them to make better health decisions and hopefully assist their peers in doing the same. Youth led education models have been associated with increased knowledge and self-efficacy as well as decreased levels of stigma and sexual risk taking behaviors (26-28). Cai et al. (26) even demonstrated a long-term benefit for a peer led education model after one year. Youth educators have also been associated with greater efficacy than adult educators in some settings. For these reasons, peer educators were chosen in our study as an important way to convey sensitive health messages to this targeted population.

Targeting the youth population eligible for the HPV vaccine is particularly challenging. This age group is beyond most mandatory vaccination programs and they are typically outside of the age for regular physician well examinations. Despite not fitting into these conventional groups, they are almost universal users of the internet, and as a result may obtain much of their health information from this source. A Pew Research study (May 2013) on teenage social media use revealed that 95% of those ages 12-17 years use the internet.

Eight in ten online teens use some kind of social media; 77% of online teens use Facebook and about one in four online teens use Twitter. Adolescents and teens are consistently accessing information online which provides an opportunity and a venue to create positive health messages in a format that appeals to them and communicate important health information. Our group of peer educators gained the desired knowledge as indicated by their survey responses and created such messages for their cohorts. They introduced messages that appealed to their interests in the form of the videos, brochures and billboards and utilized the internet, Twitter and Facebook to promote interest. During the course of the project, their participation was Tweeted, posted on Facebook and communicated to their peers, broadening the exposure of HPV and HPV vaccination into their everyday conversation.

The youth-focused creations from this project seem to resonate well with their peers as evidenced by the visits that we continually track from the website, the viewings on YouTube and by the requests from organizations for brochures for distribution to similar populations. Tailoring the message to improve education surrounding this issue is a first step. Continued efforts to maintain the website presence and the media visibility of this project are ongoing. The long term effects of this project remain to be seen. Our goal is to ultimately increase HPV vaccination uptake in our community. Increasing the HPV vaccination rates in Milwaukee, much like many other urban areas, will require continued efforts in community education, provider education and vaccine access. We need to keep tailoring our message and make health education appealing to those we are trying to reach if we are going to see real improvement.

References

[1] Koutsky L. Epidemiology of genital human papillomavirus infection. Am J Med 1997;102:3-8.

[2] Centers for Disease Control and Prevention. Human papillomavirus vaccination coverage among adolescent girls, 2007-2012, and postlicensure vaccine safety monitoring, 2006-2013 - United States. MMWR 2013;62:591-5.

[3] Dunne EF, Sternberg M, Markowitz LE, McQuillan G, Swan D, Patel S, Unger ER. Human papillomavirus (HPV) 6, 11, 16, and 18 prevalence among females in the United States--National Health And Nutrition Examination Survey, 2003-2006: opportunity to measure HPV vaccine impact? J Infect Dis 2011;204:562-5. doi: 10.1093/infdis/jir342

[4] Dunne EF, Unger ER, Sternberg M, McQuillan G, Swan DC, Patel SS, Markowitz LE. Prevalence of HPV infection among females in the United States. JAMA 2007;297:813-9. doi: 10.1001/jama.297.8.813

[5] Markowitz LE, Sternberg M, Dunne EF, McQuillan G, Unger ER. Seroprevalence of human papillomavirus types 6, 11, 16, and 18 in the United States: National Health and Nutrition Examination Survey 2003-2004. J Infect Dis 2009;200:1059-67. doi: 10.1086/604729

[6] Forman D, de Martel C, Lacey CJ, Soerjomataram I, Lortet-Tieulent J, Bruni L, Vignat J, Ferlay J, Bray F, Plummer M, Franceschi S. Global burden of human papillomavirus and related diseases. Vaccine 2012;30(Suppl 5): F12-23. doi: 10.1016/j.vaccine.2012.07.055

[7] Bosch FX, de Sanjose S. Chapter 1: Human papillomavirus and cervical cancer--burden and assessment of causality. J Natl Cancer Inst Monogr 2003;3-13.

[8] Centers for Disease Control and Prevention. Adult vaccination coverage--United States, 2010. MMWR 2012;61:66-72.

[9] Taira AV, Neukermans CP, Sanders GD. Evaluating human papillomavirus vaccination programs. Emerg Infect Dis 2004;10:1915-23. doi: 10.3201/eid1011.040222.

[10] Coupe VM, Berkhof J, Bulkmans NW, Snijders PJ, Meijer CJ. Age-dependent prevalence of 14 high-risk HPV types in the Netherlands: implications for prophylactic vaccination and screening. Br J Cancer 2008;98:646-51. doi: 10.1038/sj.bjc.6604162.

[11] Freeman HP, Wingrove BK, Center to Reduce Cancer Health Disparities (U.S.) Excess cervical cancer mortality : a marker for low access to health care in poor communities : an analysis. Rockville, MD: National Cancer Institute, Center to Reduce Cancer Health Disparities, 2005.

[12] Kahn JA, Lan D, Kahn RS (2007) Sociodemographic factors associated with high-risk human papillomavirus infection. Obstet Gynecol 2007;110:87-95. doi: 10.1097/ 01.AOG.0000266984. 23445.9c.

[13] Perkins RB, Brogly SB, Adams WG, Freund KM. Correlates of human papillomavirus vaccination rates in low-income, minority adolescents: a multicenter study. J Womens Health (Larchmt) 2012;21:813-20. doi: 10.1089/jwh.2011.3364.

[14] Downs LS, Smith JS, Scarinci I, Flowers L, Parham G. The disparity of cervical cancer in diverse populations. Gynecol Oncol 2008;109:S22-30. doi: 10.1016/j.ygyno.2008.01.003.

[15] Satterwhite CL, Torrone E, Meites E, Dunne EF, Mahajan R, Ocfemia MC, Su J, Xu F, Weinstock H. Sexually transmitted infections among US women and men: prevalence and incidence estimates, 2008. Sex Transm Dis 2013;40:187-93. doi: 10.1097/OLQ.0b013e318286bb53.

[16] Garland SM, Hernandez-Avila M, Wheeler CM, Perez G, Harper DM, Leodolter S, Tang GW, Ferris DG, Steben M, Bryan J, Taddeo FJ, Railkar R, Esser MT, Sings HL, Nelson M, Boslego J, Sattler C, Barr E, Koutsky LA. Quadrivalent vaccine against human papillomavirus to prevent anogenital diseases. N Engl J Med 2007;356:1928-43. doi: 10.1056/NEJMoa061760.

[17] Garland SM, Steben M, Sings HL, James M, Lu S, Railkar R, Barr E, Haupt RM, Joura EA. Natural history of genital warts: analysis of the placebo arm of 2 randomized phase III trials of a quadrivalent human papillomavirus (types 6, 11, 16, and 18) vaccine. J Infect Dis 2009;199:805-14. doi: 10.1086/597071.

[18] Future II Study Group. Prophylactic efficacy of a quadrivalent human papillomavirus (HPV) vaccine in women with virological evidence of HPV infection. J Infect Dis 2007; 196:1438-46. doi: 10.1086/522864.

[19] Hariri S, Markowitz LE, Dunne EF, Unger ER. Population Impact of HPV Vaccines: Summary of Early Evidence. J Adolesc Health 2013;53:679-82. doi: 10.1016/j.jadohealth.2013.09.018.

[20] Future II Study Group. Quadrivalent vaccine against human papillomavirus to prevent high-grade cervical lesions. N Engl J Med 2007;356:1915-27. doi: 10.1056/NEJMoa061741.

[21] Allen JD, Othus MK, Shelton RC, Li Y, Norman N, Tom L, del Carmen MG. Parental decision making about the HPV vaccine. Cancer Epidemiol Biomarkers Prev 2010;19: 2187-98. doi: 10.1158/1055-9965.EPI-10-0217.

[22] Conroy K, Rosenthal SL, Zimet GD, Jin Y, Bernstein DI, Glynn S, Kahn JA. Human papillomavirus vaccine uptake, predictors of vaccination, and self-reported barriers to vaccination. J Womens Health (Larchmt) 2009;18:1679-86. doi: 10.1089/jwh.2008.1329.

[23] Gowda C, Schaffer SE, Dombkowski KJ, Dempsey AF. Understanding attitudes toward adolescent vaccination and the decision-making dynamic among adolescents, parents and providers. BMC Public Health 2012;12:509. doi: 10.1186/1471-2458-12-509.

[24] Fernandez ME, Allen JD, Mistry R, Kahn JA. Integrating clinical, community, and policy perspectives on human papillomavirus vaccination. Annu Rev Public Health 2010; 31:235-52. doi: 10.1146/ annurev.publhealth.012809.103609.

[25] Centers for Disease Control and Prevention. Adult vaccination coverage--United States, 2010. MMWR 2012;61:66-72.

[26] Cai Y, Hong H, Shi R, Ye X, Xu G, Li S, Shen L. Long-term follow-up study on peer-led school-based HIV/AIDS prevention among youths in Shanghai. Int J STD AIDS 2008;19:848-50. doi: 10.1258/ijsa.2008.008129.

[27] Denison JA, Tsui S, Bratt J, Torpey K, Weaver MA, Kabaso M. Do peer educators make a difference? An evaluation of a youth-led HIV prevention model in Zambian Schools. Health Educ Res 2012;27:237-47. doi: 10.1093/her/cyr093.

[28] Ibrahim N, Rampal L, Jamil Z, Zain AM. Effectiveness of peer-led education on knowledge, attitude and risk behavior practices related to HIV among students at a Malaysian public university--a randomized controlled trial. Prev Med 2012;55:505-10. doi: 10.1016/j.ypmed.2012.09.003

In: Public Health
Editors: Rosemary M. Caron and Joav Merrick
ISBN: 978-1-63321-569-6

Chapter 9

Mobilizing a black faith community to address HIV

Magdalena Szaflarski[1,2*], Lisa M Vaughn[3], Daniel McLinden[4], Yolanda Wess[5] and Andrew Ruffner[6]

[1]Department of Sociology and Center for AIDS Research (CFAR), University of Alabama at Birmingham, Birmingham, Alabama,
[2]Department of Environmental Health, University of Cincinnati College of Medicine, Cincinnati, Ohio,
[3]Department of Pediatrics, University of Cincinnati and Division of Emergency Medicine, Cincinnati Children's Hospital Medical Center, Cincinnati, Ohio,
[4]Division of General and Community Pediatrics, Cincinnati Children's Hospital Medical Center, Cincinnati, Ohio,
[5]Department of Internal Medicine, Division of Infectious Diseases, University of Cincinnati, Cincinnati, Ohio and
[6]Department of Emergency Medicine, University of Cincinnati, Cincinnati, Ohio, US

Research that partners with community stakeholders increases contextual relevance and community buy-in and maximizes the chance for intervention success. Within a framework of an academic-community partnership, this project assessed a Black faith-community's needs and opportunities to address HIV. We used concept mapping to identify/prioritize specific HIV-related strategies that would be acceptable to congregations. Ninety stakeholders brainstormed strategies to address HIV; 21 sorted strategies into groups and rated their importance and feasibility. Multidimensional scaling and cluster analysis were applied to the sorting to produce maps that illustrated the stakeholders' conceptual thinking about HIV interventions. Of 278 responses, 93 were used in the sorting task. The visual maps represented eight clusters: church acceptance of people living with HIV; education (most feasible); mobilization and communication; church/leaders' empowerment; church involvement/collaboration; safety/HIV prevention; media outreach; and, stigma (most important). Concept mapping clarified multifaceted issues of HIV in the Black faith community. The results will guide HIV programming in congregations.

* Corresponding author: Magdalena Szaflarski, PhD, Department of Sociology, University of Alabama at Birmingham, HHB 460Q, 1720 2nd Ave S, Birmingham, AL 35294-1152, USA, Email: szaflam@uab.edu.

Introduction

Faith communities, especially African American churches, have been suggested as a key partner to address HIV (1-3). HIV, or human immunodeficiency virus, can lead to a terminal condition known as AIDS (acquired immunodeficiency syndrome). African Americans are disproportionately affected by HIV (4). The Black church (evangelical congregations predominantly made up of African American members) has been a powerful voice in communities of color, but its role in shaping HIV-risk behaviors and HIV prevention/care has been mixed (1). A national study estimated that 5.6% of U.S. congregations provide programs or activities to people living with HIV (PLWH), which were facilitated by presence of PLWH in the congregation, formal community needs assessment activities, religious tradition (Black Protestantism), and openness to gays/lesbians (5). Another study has shown that only a third of Black Protestant congregations offer HIV prevention/counseling programs (2). The literature has identified stigma linked with religious doctrines and moral positions as a key barrier to effective HIV prevention/care (6). Even churches willing to address HIV in their communities defer from discussing specific HIV-risk behaviors (7). How to tackle doctrinal stances on HIV remains unclear, but mobilization and input directly from faith leaders and faith communities in specific local contexts are emerging as useful approaches (8).

Involving community members in the process is considered as crucial to improving the success of health interventions (9). Research that partners with community stakeholders increases contextual relevance and community buy-in and therefore maximizes the chance for intervention success. As one strategy to HIV prevention, federal agencies have been funding Black churches as partners in HIV prevention (10). Most of this work has been capacity-building and HIV-related training. The development of community-based coalitions and partnerships is another effective strategy (11). Such connections have been seen as major opportunities for faith leaders to gain support and garner resources for faith communities' HIV involvement. Some faith institutions have been implementing HIV programs and services that they find acceptable within the context of their religious doctrine (12). Researchers have also begun engaging directly with faith leaders to learn about factors that facilitate or inhibit effective HIV prevention/care in at-risk communities (8).

Unfortunately, data from such studies sometimes lack rigor because traditional research and evaluation methods are difficult to implement on a large scale and in "fluid" community settings. There are also several potential barriers to implementing health programs and in particular those addressing HIV within religious settings. These include the presence of mistrust and a reciprocal lack of understanding of the values, norms, and customs between religious organizations and their partners in science, public health, or academia (13). Therefore, innovative methodologies rooted in social sciences, not widely used within public health, are urgently needed. Furthermore, demonstrations and exploratory studies need to be repeated in a broad range of environments and might even be uniquely important in areas outside of epicenters in which relatively more motivations/resources are available. Finally, community mobilization with a focus on HIV can be effective, but such interventions are most effective when they occur spontaneously and emerge directly from communities (rather than being "implemented" by an outside agent) (14). There are few studies describing programs that emerge in such "organic" fashion.

The purpose of the current study was to generate and then prioritize specific strategies to address HIV in a Black faith community. The intent was to inform the design of HIV intervention strategies based on the lived experience of the broader community of stakeholders -- providers, faith-community stakeholders (faith leaders, health ministers, and congregants), community advocates, and health researchers. Necessary here was a method that included the voice of the many and diverse perspectives of the total community and provided a process for meaning to emerge. Notably, this is the first study to examine a faith-community driven approach to HIV in the southern Midwest.

Our study

This study was conducted in Cincinnati/Hamilton County, Ohio. Hamilton County is considered a low-to-moderate HIV prevalence area with an estimated 274 per 100,000 residents living with a HIV diagnosis (15). Most (57%) of these cases are among non-Hispanic black/African Americans, and two of three Blacks with HIV in Ohio reside in Hamilton County.

A previous study has identified about 450 religious congregations in the Greater Cincinnati area, with over 100 located in the City of Cincinnati (2). About a third of Black Protestant congregations in Greater Cincinnati have offered HIV prevention/counseling programs, compared to 3-4% of other types of congregations. However, the differences in the provision of HIV programs by theology-polity have been linked to urban location, organizational resources, and broader community service (2).

The current study was conducted in the context of an academic-community partnership and a community project that involved a selected group of Black churches serving high HIV-risk neighborhoods. The program aimed to educate faith leaders about HIV and assist churches with the development of suitable, faith-based HIV stigma reduction and prevention programs. Participants in the current study were recruited from members of the faith and other community members who attended a town hall meeting organized by the academic-community partners. The target audience was faith and community leaders, health professionals, and HIV-infected or at-risk individuals. The study was approved by the University of Cincinnati Institutional Review Board.

Study design

We used *concept mapping* to generate and then prioritize specific strategies to address HIV in a Black faith community. *Concept mapping* is a mixed-method, participatory research methodology. Through brainstorming and sorting steps followed by multidimensional scaling and hierarchical cluster analysis, concept mapping results in a structured, data-driven visual representation of thoughts or ideas of a group (16). Concept mapping is an ideal participatory framework for the study of community health issues, and an extensive methodological work has demonstrated both its validity and utility. Concept mapping has been used to address substantive issues in culturally competent intervention services and health disparities (17,18). The aim of the current study was to apply concept mapping to identify contextually relevant

HIV interventions in the Black faith community and expand on prior research by involving community members in the process.

Procedure

Step 1: Brainstorming

As part of an evaluation at a community town hall meeting about HIV sponsored by our partnering community organization, attendees were asked to generate items that completed a partial statement (*focus prompt*) relevant to HIV in their community—"*To address HIV/AIDS in the Black faith community, I believe we need to....*" In concept mapping methodology, the intent of the focus prompt is to focus respondents on a specific issue, addressing HIV within the Black faith community in this case, and then ask them to provide brief responses that complete the prompt. The focus prompt was administered as part of the town hall meeting evaluation, and as such was included on a questionnaire given out at the beginning of the meeting. Attendees responded anonymously in writing with 3-5 brief responses that completed the focus prompt.

Step 2: Statement editing

Items generated in Step 1 were edited by the research team in order to reduce the number of items to a manageable set of less than 100 responses (18). The research team eliminated items not consistent with the focus prompt or items expressing similar ideas. Further editing was done for grammar and clarity of expression without altering the original meaning of the responses. The outcome of the editing process was a manageable number of items for the sorting task in Step 3.

Step 3: Sorting & rating

A smaller number of stakeholders from the same broad categories of attendees (i.e., professionals, community/church, and those personally affected by HIV) sorted the items into groups of similar ideas (19,20). Sorters were asked to identify their involvement within the HIV community (e.g., clinicians, researchers, service providers, community members, community agency, a person with HIV, and/or family member of a person with HIV. Sorters could choose to identify with more than one category. The sorters received a deck of cards and were directed to complete the sorting task. Each card contained one item generated in response to the focus prompt along with an identification number. The sorters were asked to individually sort cards into groups based on their perception of similar ideas. Next, the sorters were directed to place each group of cards into separate envelopes. On the front of the envelope, the sorters were asked to provide a label/name for each group of cards and to rate each group of cards in terms of importance and feasibility on a 5-point Likert scale.

Data analysis

Sorting data from each individual resulted in a symmetric matrix with a column and row for each of the responses. Cells in the matrix represented the intersection of each item with every other item and contained a 1 if the intersecting items were placed in the same group by the respondent or a zero if not placed in the same group. A dataset of all of the respondents' matrices was analyzed using multidimensional scaling (21) to create x,y coordinates and position the ideas as points in a two-dimensional map. Items that were often sorted together by different respondents shared a conceptual similarity in the minds of the sorters and, as a result, these items had x,y coordinates close to each other. Cluster analysis was applied to the x,y coordinates of the points to determine where boundaries could be drawn around groups of items (22). A judgment had to be made about the appropriate number of clusters because cluster analysis results in as many clusters as there are sorted responses. The goal in this interpretive process was to describe the issue in the map with as few clusters as possible but express sufficient detail. In this case, the academic-community partnership team reviewed multiple cluster solutions and determined the appropriate number of clusters. A final step was to create a label for each cluster that succinctly expressed the theme for a cluster while remaining grounded in the meaning provided by respondents. As such, the academic-community partnership team reviewed the labels used by respondents as a guide for creating final names for the clusters.

Concept maps illustrate what a group thinks about a particular issue. While the group involved in concept mapping is composed of individuals with an informed perspective, members of the group often represent multiple and diverse perspectives on the issue under consideration. An additional step that can be applied to the concept maps is to elicit the value system of the various stakeholder groups to determine the extent to which groups are in agreement. This step is accomplished by comparing value ratings provided by different stakeholder groups and then displaying and comparing the pattern of value among different groups. Termed "pattern matching" (16), the intent is to focus on the differences and similarities in the patterns of value across all of the concepts/clusters. The value that a sorter gave each group of items was assigned to all items in that grouping. The mean value for each item was then calculated across all raters, and the average value of all items in a cluster was calculated from the item means. The pattern of results was examined across all participants and within three stakeholder groups by rank-ordering the final clusters on a vertical number line for importance and feasibility. The three stakeholder groups were categorized as: 1) professionals (e.g., clinicians, researchers, service providers, etc.); 2) community (e.g., members, churches, agencies); and/or, 3) individuals personally affected by HIV (e.g., self/HIV-infected or at-risk, family members).

Findings

A total of 90 attendees to a community town hall meeting identified themselves via self-report (attendees could select more than one option) as church members/leaders associated with the project (42%), community members and members of agencies interested in addressing HIV/AIDS (45%), PLWH (8%), family member of PLWH (11%), clinician/researcher working with PLWH (20%), and other (students, visitors from another city, etc.; 13%). As part of the town hall meeting, the participants completed an evaluation that included a question about strategies to address HIV/AIDS in the Black faith community. A smaller group of stakeholders from the same broad categories (n = 21) worked individually to complete an unstructured sorting of these strategies into groups of similar ideas.

Brainstormed items

Stakeholders brainstormed a diverse set of 278 items from multiple perspectives that were relevant to addressing HIV in the Black faith community. After editing to eliminate redundant ideas and deleting items that did not respond to the focus prompt, 93 items were used in the sorting task.

Concept maps

The multidimensional scaling results (Figure 1) show how the 93 items are arranged in relation to each other; points close together represent items that the sorters considered as similar. The results also show how the 93 items coalesce into groups in the cluster analysis.

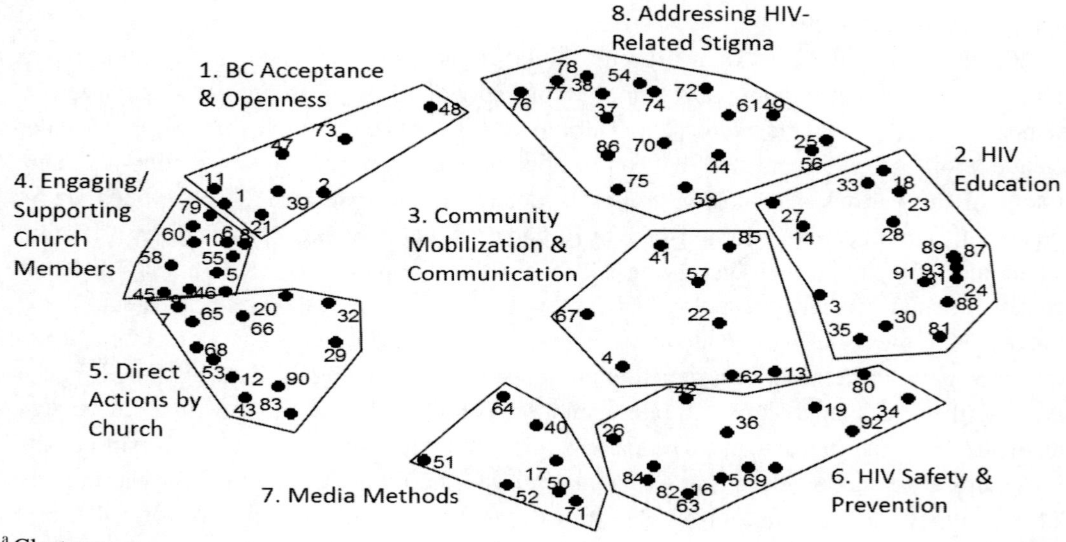

[a] Clusters:
1. Black churches' acceptance of and openness to PLWHs
2. Education about HIV among Black youth, families, and communities
3. Black community mobilization and honest communication about HIV
4. Engaging and supporting church members and leaders in talking about HIV
5. Direct actions churches can take in addressing HIV
6. Suggested strategies for HIV safety and prevention
7. Media methods to increase awareness about HIV
8. Addressing sexual and other stigmas about HIV.

Figure 1. Point and cluster map – strategies to address HIV in a Black faith community[a] (BC = Black church).

Ignoring for the moment the boundaries drawn around groups of points and the labels for those boundaries, the points alone illustrate the most detailed perspective. Based on the x,y coordinates produced by multidimensional scaling, the locations of items and the distance between items can be explored because distance between points has meaning. For example, two statements located in the lower right portion, cluster 6, are item 69, "*practice safe sex,*" which is close to item 15, "*have condoms more available*," but neither of these items are close to item 47, "*give people with HIV/AIDS love - God loves them - we should too*" located on the opposite left hand top corner of the map. The location of these points indicates that the sorters more often sorted items 69 and 15 into the same group which signifies that they thought the ideas expressed in these two items were conceptually similar. The sorters never sorted items 69 and 15 together with item 47 because the sorters saw these items as conceptually dissimilar. The multidimensional scaling routine takes the multiple data from multiple sorters and finds a single solution with best location for all points in a two-dimensional arrangement by placing the conceptually similar items closer together and the dissimilar items further apart. Because the sorting process was done individually, the sorters varied in how they organized items. For instance, items 69 and 15 may have been sorted into the same group by different sorters, but each sorter may have had different other items in the group in which 69 and 15 were placed, so these other points are nearby and still conceptually related. However, there is not complete agreement on all responses from all sorters. This illustrates a methodological nuance that is important in concept mapping -- it is not necessary to facilitate consensus in the group and thereby eliminate individual differences. Individual sorters provided their individual perspective, and the process enabled a single picture to emerge that shows where consensus exists (e.g., items 69 and 15) and where slight differences emerge (e.g., items near 69 and 15 in nearby clusters).

While understanding the nuance of point location is useful, it is also useful to see the bigger picture -- that is, applying cluster analysis to determine how multiple individual ideas represented by points coalesce into a smaller number of key concepts (*clusters*) in a map. The academic-community partnership team agreed that an eight-cluster map illustrated the key issues. Each cluster was named through a consensus process; for example, Cluster 1 was given the title, "*Black Churches' Acceptance and Openness to PLWHs*" which consisted of related responses about the church accepting PLWH (e.g., *"allow faith to evolve and progress in order to become more accepting of different lifestyles*"; Table 1).

Pattern matching

The importance and feasibility of the eight strategies were compared for each of the three stakeholder groups (i.e., professionals, community/church, and those personally affected by HIV). Keeping in mind that all items and clusters are important and to some extent feasible, pattern analysis visually orients stakeholders' priorities and beliefs about importance and feasibility. For example, across all the sorters, Cluster 8, *Addressing HIV-Related Stigma*, was rated as most important while Cluster 4, *Engaging/Supporting Church Members*, was rated as least important (Figure 2). Cluster 2, *HIV Education*, was rated as most feasible, and Cluster 1, *Black Church Acceptance and Openness*, as least feasible (Figure 2).

Table 1. Example responses in each cluster

Cluster 1: Black churches' acceptance of and openness to people living with HIV (PLWH) *1. Help the churches become more accepting of men that have sex with men* *2. Allow faith to evolve and progress in order to become more accepting of different lifestyles* *21. Address the issue in church - we know abstinence is not the message, so let's get real*
Cluster 2: Education about HIV among Black youth, families, and communities *30. Educate the public on the risks involved with unprotected sex* *89. Get young people talking about HIV/AIDS and educate them* *14. Acknowledge that this epidemic is impacting our community*
Cluster 3: Black community mobilization and honest communication about HIV *13. Mobilize community to talk about the issue (prevention, social and population behaviors)* *57. Encourage HIV/AIDS at home conversations with families or at family reunions* *85. Discuss contextual factors that affect African American women and female adolescents such as SES, negotiation skills, etc.*
Cluster 4: Engaging and supporting church members and leaders in talking about HIV *8. For the church leadership to proclaim their support of HIV/AIDS prevention and pass this on to their congregations* *46. Listen to members of the church and how they deal with HIV/AIDS* *79. Address it openly and lovingly in church - no shame! Within the church (pastor and family included)*
Cluster 5: Direct actions churches can take in addressing HIV *12. Have more churches collaborating on prevention/education activities* *53. Work it through our health ministry* *83. Offer HIV testing at the church*
Cluster 6: Suggested strategies for HIV safety and prevention *16. Prevent - offer contraception as opposed to just abstinence* *69. Practice safe sex* *92. Develop interesting ways to engage youth and encourage youth testing (events, concerts, famous people endorsements)*
Cluster 7: Media methods to increase awareness about HIV *50. TV- radio - public announcements* *51. Upgrade marketing efforts in the faith initiative every sermon - billboards – public service announcements - radio announcements Sunday* *71. Hit social media, that's where the youth reside*
Cluster 8: Addressing sexual and other stigmas about HIV *25. Take it out of the closet and educate that HIV/AIDS is now a heterosexual problem* *37. Openly discuss issues pertaining to the gay Black community* *76. Address the sense of homophobia/stigma that is so often attached to feelings regarding homosexuality in this community*

Pattern analysis was also used to explore the beliefs about importance and feasibility within stakeholder groups. For example, the professionals rated Cluster 8, *Addressing HIV-Related Stigma*, as most important and Cluster 5, *Direct Actions by Church*, as least important (Figure 3). They rated Cluster 6, *HIV Safety & Prevention*, as the most feasible and Cluster 1, *Black Church Acceptance and Openness*, as the least feasible strategy. The community group rated Cluster 3, *Community Mobilization & Communication*, as most important and Cluster 5, *Direct Actions by Church*, as least important (Figure 4). The community group rated Cluster 2, *HIV Education*, as most feasible and Cluster 1, *Black Church Acceptance and Openness*, as least feasible. Finally, the group personally affected by HIV rated Cluster 6, *HIV Safety & Prevention*, as most important while Cluster 4, *Engaging/ Supporting Church Members*, was rated as least important (Figure 5). For those personally affected by HIV, Cluster 8, *Addressing HIV-Related Stigma*, was rated as most feasible, and Cluster 1, *Black Church Acceptance and Openness*, was rated as least feasible.

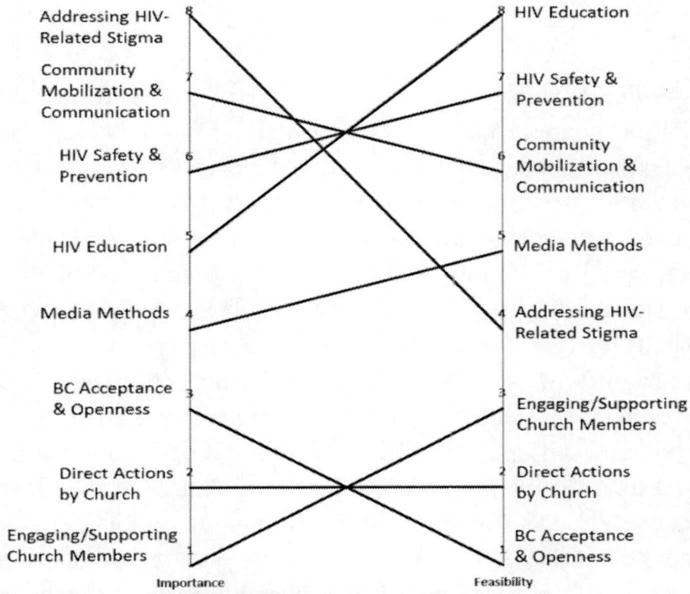

[a] Higher values indicate greater importance and greater feasibility

[b] Professionals, community, and individuals personally affected by HIV (i.e., HIV-infected and at-risk individuals; family/friends of people living with HIV [PLWH]).

Figure 2. Pattern matching of rank-ordered clusters by importance and feasibility[a]: all sorters[b] (BC = Black church).

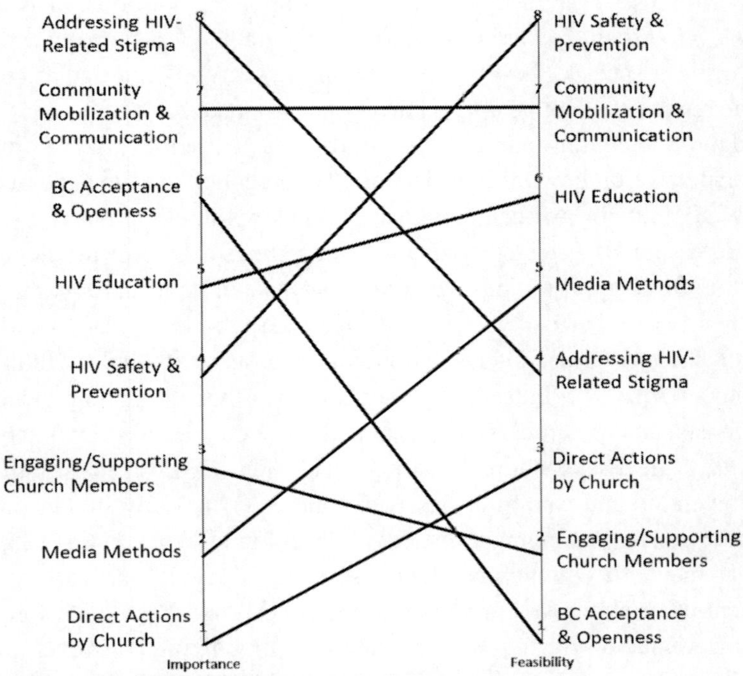

[a] Higher values indicate greater importance and greater feasibility.

Figure 3. Pattern matching of rank-ordered clusters by importance and feasibility[a]: professionals (BC = Black church).

Discussion

There is increasing interest and research activity on African American faith community's involvement in HIV prevention. Concept mapping was used in the current study to identify and prioritize contextually relevant HIV-related strategies within a local Black faith community. Community-based approaches are recognized for their utility in disparities reduction efforts, due to their emphasis on inclusion of those communities most directly affected by the disparity to identify problems and potential solutions. Without these perspectives, professionals in public health, HIV treatment, and research fields may not identify the complexity of issues that could have an impact on outcomes. To develop the concept maps, we sought to obtain diverse perspectives on faith-based HIV prevention by including church members and leaders who were currently involved in an HIV prevention project, PLWH and their family members, HIV clinicians/researchers, and other community members who had expressed interest through their attendance at a community town hall meeting on HIV in the African American faith community. In doing so, we were able to represent views from both inside and outside of the social systems that might be involved in a community response to HIV. By maximizing the diversity of the respondents, the resulting concept maps can be placed in the context of stakeholders' collective experience and values.

Like any methodology, concept mapping has limitations including nonrandom sampling, small sample size, and the time and labor-intensive process required to involve multiple stakeholders. However, concept mapping provides researchers and practitioners with a unique, participatory data collection and intervention design process that allows for individual-level responses (brainstorming) and group-level wisdom (sorting and data analysis). In addition, this study was specific to one geographic location and a selected group of individuals within a specific faith community and that group's particular concerns; thus, the content of the results may not be applicable to other contexts.

These limitations notwithstanding, this study offers useful insights into the faith community's perspective on how faith leaders and congregations can engage in public health efforts to address HIV among African Americans. One key finding in our study was the high importance of addressing HIV-related stigma in faith settings and some problems with (lower feasibility of) this strategy. Previous research has shown that faith communities have frequently shunned persons at risk of HIV, such as men who have sex with men and drug users, because of strict doctrinal interpretations of religious texts and a culture of silence, stigma, and homophobia (1). Indeed, representatives of various groups, including faith leaders, HIV activists, and researchers, have claimed for over a decade that homophobia *is* the key factor blocking the Black church's response to HIV (23,24). These attitudes hinder effective HIV prevention and care in at-risk communities (10). Many studies have identified stigma as a specific barrier to congregational involvement in HIV prevention (25).

The fact that the faith community in our study considered addressing stigma as less feasible than some other strategies suggests that the Black church is not as well equipped to tackle HIV stigma versus delivering HIV education or mobilizing. However, although HIV stigma is typically an issue within conservative churches, some denominations and churches have been able to address stigma despite conservative theologies (25). For example, congregations can donate resources to support HIV-related programs, such as condom distribution and clean needle exchanges, as part of their service mission, without engaging in such activities directly (26). Other congregations simply follow their ideology of welcoming *all* people, regardless of their lifestyles (e.g., homo-/bi-sexuality) or disease (e.g., HIV) states or risks (27). Research shows that presence of PLWH in the congregation and openness to gays/lesbians, among other factors, helps to enhance congregational HIV programming (5).

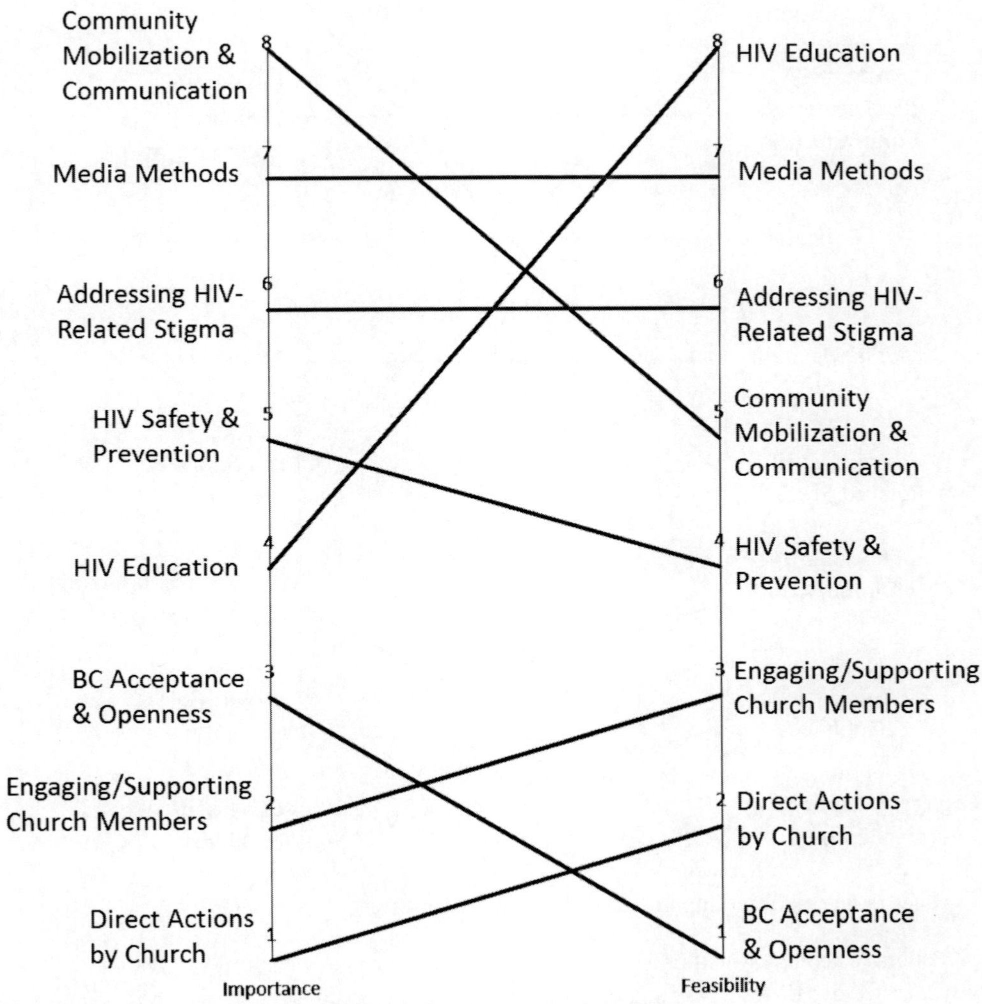

[a] Higher values indicate greater importance and greater feasibility.

Figure 4. Pattern matching of rank-ordered clusters by importance and feasibility[a]: community (BC = Black church).

In our study, addressing stigma and community mobilization were identified as distinct strategies (i.e., different clusters). However, the literature suggests that they are more intertwined. For example, Tyrell and colleagues (28) propose that the faith community history of shaming and blaming deters HIV prevention efforts, and the way to address this is by engaging faith leaders who are historically the community mobilizers in the Black community. The impact of stigma on behaviors and self-perceptions of PLWH is important because those who are stigmatized are less likely to display health-seeking behavior. Stigma can make people less likely to seek an HIV test, less likely to disclose HIV status if they are positive, and more likely to engage in high-risk sexual activities (28), further emphasizing the importance of our study in aiding the Black church in choosing interventions that can lessen HIV-related stigma.

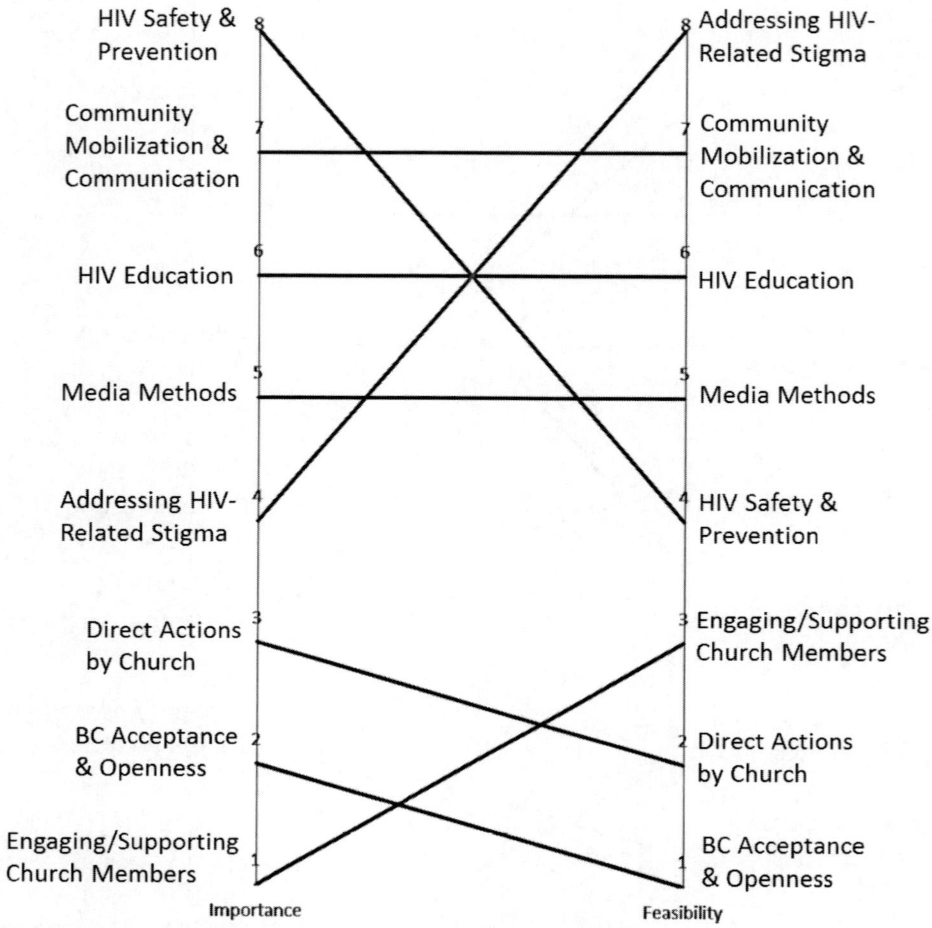

[a] Higher values indicate greater importance and greater feasibility.

Figure 5. Pattern matching of rank-ordered clusters by importance and feasibility[a]: individuals personally affected by HIV (BC = Black church).

Interestingly, people affected by HIV rated tackling stigma lower in importance than the other groups in our study while they rated this strategy as the most feasible. One potential explanation for such views is the perception that attitude change does not require resources. Another explanation could be that people affected by HIV often participate in settings that welcome them, and stigma appears not to be a significant problem in those settings. Further research will need to clarify the perspectives of people affected by HIV on the stigma problem within faith communities.

Another cluster of strategies proposed by the faith community in our study focused on the need for community outreach. Previous research has shown that faith leaders and congregations are often unaware of the extent of the HIV epidemic in their surrounding communities and thus feel no sense of need or urgency (25). If an intervention can rectify this issue, churches may be willing to engage in HIV-related activities. For example, in one project, data were presented to churches on various health problems, including HIV, in the geographic communities surrounding the churches, and the congregations chose themselves to target HIV and youth sexual risk behaviors in their health programming (29). Research at the national level shows that formal community HIV-related needs assessments facilitate the provision of HIV programming (5). Raising awareness through dissemination of data about the local epidemic is also one strategy to change attitudes about and increase compassion for persons with or at high risk of HIV in the faith communities (30).

Our data suggest that faith-community mobilization is a key component of HIV-related community outreach and that supporting the Black faith community mobilization efforts is highly feasible as well as highly important. Many Black churches around the country have taken a stance on homophobia and have led efforts locally and nationally to address HIV stigma, for example, the Trinity United Church of Christ, a Black-mega church; the Balm in Gilead, an organization based in New York City that has championed HIV awareness and intervention for three decades; the Regional AIDS Interfaith Network in North Carolina; and, Unity Fellowship Churches based in several large metropolitan areas (24,31). Partnerships between faith-based, public health, and academic institutions have emerged all across the country. Some of these coalitions engage large numbers of churches; for example, a Michigan program engaged more than 40 congregations (32). The evidence suggests that with resources and multiple stakeholders at the table, faith-based community outreach is highly feasible. Although sustainability of programs remains limited, community-driven interventions have unique potential vis-à-vis other types of interventions because they capitalize on strengths of communities and attain community trust needed to address HIV (32).

The findings from our study also indicate the high importance and feasibility of faith-based educational and media campaigns. The use of faith communities as both agents and target audiences in the dissemination of HIV-related information and messages is innovative and can supplement traditional educational and media approaches. The need for HIV safety and prevention knowledge dissemination in this faith community was rated among the top three items in importance and feasibility. However, the literature suggests that only certain messages tend to be acceptable in faith-based settings. For example, one study showed that faith leaders have a strong preference for abstinence-based sex education, and they are not willing to discuss specific behaviors associated with HIV transmission (7). Furthermore, engaging and supporting church members in discussing HIV at the congregational forum were rated low in importance and feasibility among our community stakeholders. These findings indicate limited readiness of this community to address the faith/doctrinal aspects related to HIV. The community partners in our project repeatedly stressed the importance of "meeting the churches where they are" -- that is, offering congregations options for HIV involvement that would not compromise or negate their religious doctrine.

In our sample, respondents were able to identify and had fair levels of agreement about specific strategies to address HIV within the Black church, as evidenced by content areas involved in the clusters. Next steps include forming action groups at the participating churches composed of church members who are interested in developing specific interventions to address HIV based on the identified clusters. The eight-cluster concept maps will be used to guide the process and ensure that all viewpoints are considered, rather than the individual church or one group of stakeholders having a dominant voice. Specific brainstormed responses underlying the clusters can be consulted alongside existing models and research about how to best address HIV within this Black faith community. The concept maps can also facilitate considerations of various levels which need to be addressed (e.g., church, broader community, society) within the design of an HIV-related intervention or program.

The eight clusters identified in this study can serve as a roadmap for an improved understanding of the types of HIV approaches that are most promising and those that are less likely to be acceptable to this Black faith community for implementation. Without input from and inclusion of all relevant stakeholders, interventions may be void of the lived experience and daily lives of those affected. Efforts to eliminate or reduce HIV-related disparities must involve local communities and consider their views, thereby increasing individual and community ability to address the existing concerns in the community.

Acknowledgments

The project described was supported by the National Center for Research Resources and the National Center for Advancing Translational Sciences, National Institutes of Health, through Grant 8 UL1 TR000077-05. Preliminary work for this project was supported by the *Eunice Kennedy Shriver* National Institute of Child Health and Human Development, through Grant 5R21HD050137-02. The content is solely the responsibility of the authors and does not necessarily represent the official views of the National Institutes of Health. Specifically, the project was funded through a Community Health Grant from the University of Cincinnati Center for Clinical and Translational Science and Training (CCTST). The grantee was *IV-CHARIS*, a faith-based non-profit HIV service agency in Cincinnati, Ohio. Dr. Szaflarski and Dr. Vaughn were the academic co-principal investigators on the project. This research was presented at the University of Alabama at Birmingham 8th Annual Health Disparities Research Symposium, where it received the Charles Barkley Health Disparities Investigator 1st Place (Oral Presentation) Award from the Minority Health Disparities Research Center.

We thank the following collaborators for their contributions: Ms. Mamie Harris, CDCA, and Camisha Chambers, BA of *IV-CHARIS*, Cincinnati, Ohio, for leading the community mobilization and program implementation effort and assistance with data collection; Nancy Peter, BA of the University of Cincinnati Local Performance Site, Pennsylvania/MidAtlantic AIDS Education and Training Center (PAMAAETC), for her assistance with educational programming and partnership-building activities; Chandra Smith, MSW, LISW and the Cincinnati Queen Chapter of Delta Sigma Theta Sorority, Inc. for their community mobilization efforts and in-kind support; and, LaSharon Mosley, PhD for assistance with data design and collection. Also, special thanks to the CCTST leaders: Joel Tsevat, MD, MPH, for senior advice and research ethics support, and Monica Mitchell, PhD, for linking us with the CCTST Community Engagement Core and its resources. We also thank P. Neal Ritchey, PhD for guidance on coalition-building and program evaluation; Ruchi Bawa, MPH for research assistance at the onset of the project; Cathy Siemer (PAMAAETC) for administrative support; and, Teresa Smith, BA (CCTST) for grant-related assistance.

Last, but not least, we would like to acknowledge and commend the following congregations and faith leaders for their participation in the project and in-kind support (e.g., meeting space): Zion Global Ministries – Pastor Freddie T. Piphus; Gaines United Methodist

Church – Pastor Curnell Graham; St. Mark Missionary Baptist Church – Pastor Dr. Cecil Ferrell; Corinthian Baptist Church – Pastor KZ Smith; New Prospect Baptist Church – Pastor Damon Lynch III; Lincoln Heights Missionary Baptist Church – Pastor Dr. Elliott Cuff; Turning Point Church of Zion – Pastor James Bready; Light of the World Ministries – Pastor Mike Scruggs; St. Mark A.M.E. Zion - Pastor Jermaine Armor; Bethel Baptist Church - Pastor Wayne Davis; Tryed Stone New Beginnings - Pastor Jerry Culbreth; Inspirational Baptist Church - Pastor Victor Couzens; World Outreach Christian Center - Pastor Gregory Chandler; and, Second Trinity Church - Pastor Kenneth Bibb.

References

[1] Sutton MY, Parks CP. HIV/AIDS prevention, faith, and spirituality among Black/African American and Latino communities in the United States: strengthening scientific faith-based efforts to shift the course of the epidemic and reduce HIV-related health disparities. J Relig Health 2013;52(2):514-30.

[2] Szaflarski M, Ritchey PN, Jacobson CJ, Williams RH, Baumann Grau A, Meganathan K, et al. Faith-based HIV prevention and counseling programs: findings from the Cincinnati Census of Religious Congregations. AIDS Behav 2013;17:1839-54.

[3] Szaflarski, M. Spirituality and religion among HIV-infected individuals. Curr HIV/AIDS Rep 2013;10(4):324-32.

[4] Centers for Disease Control and Prevention. HIV among African Americans. 2013. URL: http://www.cdc.gov/hiv/pdf/risk_HIV_AfricanAmericans.pdf

[5] Frenk SM, Trinitapoli J. U.S. congregations' provision of programs or activities for people living with HIV/AIDS. AIDS Behav 2013;17(5):1829-38.

[6] Williams JK, Wyatt GE, Wingood G. The four Cs of HIV prevention with African Americans: crisis, condoms, culture, and community. Curr HIV/AIDS Rep 2010;7(4):185-93.

[7] Francis SA, Lam WK, Cance JD, Hogan VK. What's the 411? Assessing the feasibility of providing African American adolescents with HIV/AIDS prevention education in a faith-based setting. J Relig Health 2009;48(2):164-77.

[8] Nunn A, Cornwall A, Chute N, Sanders J, Thomas G, James G, et al. Keeping the faith: African American faith leaders' perspectives and recommendations for reducing racial disparities in HIV/AIDS infection. PloS One 2012;7(5):e36172.

[9] Minkler M, Wallerstein N. Community-based participatory research for health: from process to outcomes, 2nd ed. San Francisco, CA: Jossey-Bass, 2008.

[10] Eke AN, Wilkes AL, Gaiter J. Organized religion and the fight against HIV/AIDS in the black community: the role of the Black Church. In: McCree DH, ed. African Americans and HIV/AIDS: understanding and addressing the epidemic. New York: Springer, 2010:53-68.

[11] Centers for Disease Control and Prevention. CDC executive summary: CDC consultation on faith and HIV prevention. 2006. URL: http://www.cdc.gov/hiv//resources/other/PDF/faith.pdf

[12] Derose KP, Mendel PJ, Palar K, Kanouse DE, Bluthenthal RN, Castaneda LW, et al. Religious congregations' involvement in HIV: a case study approach. AIDS Behav 2011;15(6):1220-32.

[13] Campbell MK, Hudson MA, Resnicow K, Blakeney N, Paxton A, Baskin M. Church-based health promotion interventions: evidence and lessons learned. Ann Rev Public Health 2007;28:213-34.

[14] Blankenship KM, Friedman SR, Dworkin S, Mantell JE. Structural interventions: concepts, challenges and opportunities for research. J Urban Health 2006;83(1):59-72.

[15] Ohio Department of Health. HIV/AIDS integrated epidemiological profile for Ohio: 2011 edition. Columbus, OH: Ohio Department of Health, 2012.

[16] Trochim WMK, Kane M. Concept mapping: an introduction to structured conceptualization in health care. Int J Qual Health Care 2005;17(3):187-91.

[17] Jackson KM, Trochim WMK. Concept mapping as an alternative approach for the analysis of open-ended survey responses. Organ Res Meth 2002;5(4):307-36.

[18] Vaughn LM, Jacquez, F, McLinden, D. The use of concept mapping to identify community-driven intervention strategies for physical and mental health. Health Promot Pract 2013:14(5):675-85.

[19] Rosenberg S, Moonja Park K. The method of sorting as a data gathering procedure in multivariate research. Multivar Behav Res 1975;10(4):489-502.

[20] Weller SC, Romney AK. Systematic data collection. Newbury Park, CA: Sage, 1988.

[21] de Leeuw J, Mair P. Multidimensional scaling using majorization: SMACOF in R. J Stat Softw 2009;31(3):1-30.

[22] Kane M, Trochim WMK. Concept mapping for planning and evaluation. Thousand Oaks: Sage, 2007.

[23] Fullilove MT, Fullilove RE. Stigma as an obstacle to AIDS action: the case of the African American community. Am Behav Sci 1999;42(7):1117-29.

[24] Ward EG. Homophobia, hypermasculinity and the US black church. Cult Health Sex 2005;7(5):493-504.

[25] Williams MV, Palar K, Derose KP. Congregation-based programs to address HIV/AIDS: elements of successful implementation. J Urban Health 2011;88(3):517-32.

[26] Koch JR, Beckley RE. Under the radar: AIDS ministry in the bible belt. Rev Relig Res 2006;47(4):393-408.

[27] Leong P. Religion, flesh, and blood: re-creating religious culture in the context of HIV/AIDS. Sociol Relig 2006;67(3):295-311.

[28] Tyrell CO, Klein SJ, Gieryic SM, Devore BS, Cooper JG, Tesoriero JM. Early results of a statewide initiative to involve faith communities in HIV prevention. J Public Health Manag Pract 2008;14(5):429-36.

[29] Kruger DJ, Lewis Y, Schlemmer E. Mapping a message for faith leaders: encouraging community health promotion with local health data. Health Promot Pract 2010;11(6):837-44.

[30] Bluthenthal RN, Palar K, Mendel P, Kanouse DE, Corbin DE, Derose KP. Attitudes and beliefs related to HIV/AIDS in urban religious congregations: barriers and opportunities for HIV-related interventions. Soc Sci Med 2012;74(10):1520-7.

[31] Cohen C. The boundaries of Blackness: AIDS and the breakdown of Black politics. Chicago: University of Chicago Press, 1999.

[32] Griffith DM, Pichon LC, Campbell B, Allen JO. YOUR Blessed Health: a faith-based CBPR approach to addressing HIV/AIDS among African Americans. AIDS Educ Prev 2010;22(3):203-17.

In: Public Health
Editors: Rosemary M. Caron and Joav Merrick

ISBN: 978-1-63321-569-6

Chapter 10

Public health and academic partners and how to address infant mortality

Jennifer Mooney*, PhD[1], Farrah Jacquez, PhD[2] and William Scott[1]
[1]Reproductive Health and Wellness Program, Maternal and Infant Health Division, Cincinnati Health Department and [2]Department of Psychology, University of Cincinnati, Cincinnati, Ohio, US

A partnership between a sociologist at a public health department and a psychologist at a university collaborated on a service learning project that addressed the high infant mortality rate in the region. By addressing unintended teen pregnancy and by examining factors contributing to fetal or infant loss, the partnership provided practicum students with opportunities to use the scientific method to examine infant mortality and disseminate findings to local stakeholders. The public health department benefited through additional workforce power in unbiased data analysis and reporting of results, which led to program enhancement. The students benefited by conducting translational research salient to our community. Strategies for building sustainable partnerships are discussed.

Introduction

Infant mortality, in a public health sense, serves as a gauge of overall community health and is defined as the death of an infant before his or her first birthday. The national infant mortality rate per one thousand births in the United States is 6.06 – a rate much higher than that in other developed countries (1). Although infant mortality in the United States has declined in recent years (1), infant death in the Cincinnati-Hamilton County region of Ohio is nearly triple the Healthy People 2010 goal and double the national average (1,2). Infant mortality has recently evolved to epidemic status in Cincinnati, although the issue has not

* Correspondence: Jennifer Mooney, PhD, Director, Reproductive Health and Wellness Program, Maternal and Infant Health Division, Cincinnati Health Department, 3101 Burnet Avenue, Cincinnati, Ohio 45229, United States. E-mail: jennifer.mooney@cincinnati-oh.gov.

affected all racial groups equally. At a rate of 17.8 deaths per 1000 births, African Americans have more than double the infant mortality rate of White residents (3-5). Considering the elevated overall infant mortality rate and the striking racial disparity in infant deaths, social and medical scientists are trying to untangle the web of factors that contribute to negative birth outcomes. Given the complexity of such disparities, interdisciplinary collaboration between public health and academic partners provides a unique way to dissect health concerns with greater rigor and objectivity.

Social determinants of infant mortality

The Cincinnati Health Department and its partnering social service agencies and community organizations have prioritized infant mortality as the key public health issue in our area and have started to investigate the unique social determinants of infant mortality in Cincinnati. Perhaps partially due to the fragmented landscape of health services for women in our area, understanding the perinatal risks for both women and their babies is multifaceted and therefore quite complicated. Unintended pregnancy, for instance, is documented as an indicator of poor birth outcomes (6). However, in a largely Catholic hospital delivery system, few post-partum women are discharged from the delivery hospital with contraception, thereby increasing the chances that these women might become pregnant before the recommended time of at least eighteen months post-delivery.

Pregnancy intention has been documented as a correlate of infant mortality, in that family planning can reduce infant mortality (7). Teen mothers are more likely to experience unintentional pregnancies, thereby increasing risks for adverse health outcomes. Proper prevention of unwanted pregnancy is also affected by the sociopolitical landscape. Research shows that young mothers with unwanted pregnancies are more likely to miss important prenatal visits (8), engage in risky behavior such as smoking or illicit drug use during pregnancy (9), and are more likely to suffer from postpartum depression than adult mothers who plan pregnancy (10). It has also been found that teen mothers often have poorer physical and mental health outcomes later in life than women who did not experience teen motherhood (11).

When attempting to promote optimal infant health and avoid mortality, social service agents and healthcare professionals tend to focus on those factors in which they have expertise. Primary care physicians may be more concerned with weight gain and hypertension as correlates of poor birth outcomes. Social workers may be more likely to contribute high infant mortality rates to domestic issues or access to social services. Obstetricians might focus on participation in prenatal healthcare as the primary target for intervention. In order to address the complex problem of infant mortality, collaboration among diverse stakeholders with varying skill sets and subjectivities is essential. Essentially, untangling the web of human behaviors that led to a pregnancy and ultimately a birth involves both social and medical perspectives.

University-public health department partnership

A truly successful partnership is considered to be a pooling of resources where each partner exercises power in decision-making (12). Research also suggests that successful collaboration be predicated on common interests and goals, mutual cooperation and shared responsibility, and expected mutual benefit (13). From a public health perspective, effective collaboration can be executed through evidence-based research that bridges the gaps between research, practice, and policy. Implementing a public health program through evidence-based research allows the data to inform the program policies and allows for replication of the program. Embracing a solid research foundation for government spending is vital for maximizing public health dollars; at the same time, the logistical barriers of conducting research in real-world programs must be understood by academic researchers (4). Prior examination of the relationship between research and policy has suggested that research must be rigorous, policy must be legitimate, acceptable, and socially relevant, and practice must have applicability (4). While seemingly fundamental, these guidelines for successful partnerships can prove quite challenging when the partnership demands energy and time above and beyond the scope of work for the collaborating partners.

Collaboration between academia and public health is not a new concept. Some partnerships are sustainable and others are time limited. For instance, when Connecticut experienced an increase of a vancomycin-resistant enterococci (VRE) incidence, registered nurses enrolled in a master's of science of nursing program collaborated with the physicians and epidemiologists of the Department of Public Health to address the issue (14). The emergency preparedness team found the resources necessary to address an epidemic and the nursing students were able to apply their skills to address an acute issue in the community. More sustainable academic-public health partnerships do not revolve around a single public health issue, have a longer developmental period, and tend to have less immediate results. For instance, Georgia's Fulton County Sickness Prevention Achieved through Regional Collaboration (SPARC) is a collaborative effort between public, nonprofit, and public health stakeholders to provide clinic-based preventive care to senior citizens. Over time, the dynamic collaboration has been flexible in changing strategies to meet its overall mission and has and scored high when evaluated for program effectiveness (12).

Like all partnerships, ideal university-public health partnerships are formed with the expectations of mutual benefits. Academic partnerships with public health departments can directly benefit students by guiding the career path of students toward public health; therefore, students gain education and experience while public health departments build their future workforce. Previous literature has demonstrated that partnerships have been beneficial for student nurses who were naïve to nursing within the public health system until practicums opened for them to gain experience (15). Students gain access to resources offered by public health partnerships and can undertake training in order to shape their expertise and professional training (3). Based on their participation in public health activities as undergraduates, students are more likely to choose that path post-graduation (3).

The marriage of public health and academic research benefits public health departments by increasing scientific rigor of public health program efforts. For instance, partnerships with universities help protect against external bias because universities are less likely to have a conflict of interest. Financial incentives of outside parties, such as the pharmaceutical industry, play less into the direction of policy making when a non-biased academic institution is utilized instead as a partner (16). In addition, university-based partners (particularly students) have the benefit of naivety when collaborating in public health research. Unlike the hard-working public professionals who provide programming efforts and are highly invested in results, universities and students serve as an outside party with the goal of objectivity.

Barriers to healthy partnerships have been identified as the breakup of previously established networks and a risk of cost cutting on public health interventions that were previously shown to be effective (17). Partnerships should be manageable and when they are built on similar principles, values, and goals, the likelihood of sustainability increases (13).

Because public health is multidisciplinary, the opportunities for collaboration with academic partners are vast. However, the structure of the Cincinnati public health department employs methods that include surveillance, assessment, disease prevention, health education, and assuring access to public health services (18). With the many demands from the local public health system and the variety of skillsets of its employees, finding research minded individuals for academics to partner with could be challenging. The mission of academia, after all, is to provide unbiased guidance for tomorrow's leaders through education, peer review, and scientific rigor. The collaboration discussed in this paper holds that partnerships based on science and utilization of the naivety of research students is beneficial to public health epidemiology.

The goals of this project are to offer an effective strategy for building a sustainable university-public health partnership. The partnership we describe was established with careful planning, execution, and monitoring in part due to the sensitive nature of infant mortality as a subject matter. As a result of the collaboration, two successful public health projects targeting infant mortality were implemented. Each project provided benefits to both partners, generated useful knowledge for enhancing public health programs, and provided students with an active learning environment. We will discuss the partners, the process of establishing the partnership, the results of the collaboration, and the benefits and challenges of university-public health partnerships.

Our project

We describe a university-public health department partnership to address infant mortality. The participants in the collaboration are the Cincinnati Health Department and the University of Cincinnati psychology capstone course.

Cincinnati Health Department

The first author, a sociologist at the CHD, serves as the public health partner in our university-health department collaboration. Within the division of Maternal and Infant Health at the CHD, Dr. Mooney oversees the data team of the Fetal and Infant Mortality Review (FIMR) program and is the director for the Cincinnati Hamilton County Reproductive Health and Wellness Program (RHWP), operating in CHD's six federally qualified health centers. FIMR and RHWP address infant mortality in two unique ways. The FIMR program examines fetal and infant death through a case review process while the RHWP prevents unintended pregnancy through family planning and contraception.

Fetal and Infant Mortality Review (FIMR)

FIMR serves women and families with a fetal or infant loss, is operated from the Cincinnati and Hamilton County Health Departments, and is intended to enhance the Greater Cincinnati community. Women and families are provided the opportunity to share the story of their baby's death with a trained interviewer, facilitating the grief process and providing opportunities for education and referrals. Traditionally, the FIMR process required the case review team to review individual level interview data and vital statistics to assess where system enhancements can be made. Prior to the current partnership, FIMR had never undergone any rigorous data analysis on the aggregate level. Suggestions to the community action team were usually made on a case-by-case basis. Trends were not mapped, nor were community level analyses conducted.

Reproductive Health & Wellness Program (RHWP)

The RHWP commenced in 2012 and serves the entire Hamilton County, although the majority of eligible patients live in Cincinnati proper. Federally funded through Title X, the RHWP is designed to improve the health and well-being of women, men, and children by improving their access to preventative and primary health care, promoting healthy behaviors and encouraging the establishment of a reproductive life plan. Patients are provided reproductive health care, including a wide variety of contraception, on a sliding scale. Rigorous program evaluation is ongoing for clinical visits although analysis on the existing RHWP outreach spinoffs is much needed. Outreach drives the mission of the clinical program and therefore, data analysis is critical.

University of Cincinnati Psychology Capstone Course

The academic partner in our university-health department partnership (second author) is a professor in the psychology department at the University of Cincinnati whose research focuses on community approaches to health disparities. Dr. Jacquez teaches the senior psychology capstone course, a class designed to provide advanced undergraduates with a culminating experience applying the knowledge and skills they acquired while progressing through the psychology major. Approximately 20 senior psychology students are enrolled in the capstone course each semester. Unlike other capstone options within the psychology department, students enrolled in this capstone participate in a service-learning experience designed to translate research skills into real-world settings. The goal of this course is for students to understand how psychological research can be used to address locally relevant questions about child health. By working with a community agency, students have the opportunity to see how research is crucial to solving real world problems. In addition, students provide a meaningful, much-needed contribution to our understanding of infant mortality in Cincinnati.

The capstone course is designed to provide advanced undergraduates with learning opportunities that make real community impact. Although service-learning projects each semester are unique, the goals of the course are fairly consistent. Students must demonstrate competency in a set of research skills, including reviewing academic literature, analyzing data, interpreting data in ways that will be meaningful to community partners, and writing research reports. Students collaborate directly with the public health partner throughout the semester, including off-site visits to the Cincinnati Health Department to learn more about programs and present results. Since the partnership between the CHD and the UC capstone course began approximately two years ago, three semesters of capstone students have had the opportunity to participate in service learning experiences directly or indirectly addressing infant mortality.

The current partnership

The purpose of collaboration is to pool the resources of academic partners (a clinical psychologist and advanced undergraduate psychology students) and public health partners (a sociologist and public health department staff) to address infant mortality in a way that progresses both (1) the program trajectory in public health, and (2) the pedagogy of psychology capstone students. Both supervising partners share similar interests and have backgrounds in research; particularly experimental design, human subjects protection, data integrity, and translation of findings to practice. In addition, both academic and community partners served on the Fetal and Infant Mortality Review (FIMR) case review team and are both interested in identifying and developing interventions to address the social determinants of infant mortality.

The current partnership was formed to address the often overlooked social determinants of health as contributors to the region's high infant mortality rate. We will present two examples of projects our partnership has completed: first, an in-depth analysis of FIMR interviews, and second, an evaluation of a program serving teens seeking reproductive health care in schools. Both semester long service-learning projects were designed to help 1) senior psychology students complete their capstones, 2) the CHD obtain quality data that informs program development, and 3) pave an avenue for further collaboration. Several logistical considerations have been made during each semester of collaboration. A "Not Human Subjects" exemption form was submitted to the Institutional Review Board (IRB) at the University as to exempt the project from being defined as "research." Project findings were to be used internally rather than shared with the public, and data was de-identified. Students were mandated to successfully complete a Collaborative Institutional Training Initiative (CITI) human subjects training course prior to beginning the project. Consent was received from the CHD and a Memorandum of Understanding (MOU) was on file prior to collaboration.

In each example project presented, the academic and community partner worked together closely when designing the course to plan activities that met both CHD and student needs. For instance, the syllabus was designed by both academic and community partners to ensure that outcomes of class activities could directly benefit CHD programs. The academic partner incorporated the community partner into elements of the classroom, added her name to the course syllabus as the Community Professor, and held class at the CHD on occasion so students might more easily translate their experience into real world practice. Finally, at the end of each project, students presented their written report in person to relevant stakeholders at the CHD.

Findings

Project #1: Fetal and Infant Mortality Review (FIMR)

The goal of the FIMR project was to utilize the research skills of capstone students to identify social determinants of health within existing FIMR data. Using qualitative methods and collaboratively taught by both academic and community partners, capstone students analyzed transcripts of FIMR interviews with mothers who had lost an infant. FIMR interviews contain a wealth of information about the life and healthcare experiences of women who experience a fetal/infant loss; however, until this partnership, the data had not undergone rigorous qualitative and quantitative analysis. The three objectives of the service learning project were 1) to identify themes common among mothers who experienced infant loss; 2) to describe how often mothers reported these themes; and 3) to identify significant relationships between demographic variables and themes. Themes derived from this project were to be used by FIMR to create recommendations for interventions.

The FIMR project had significant benefits for both the students and the health department. Students learned methods for conducting both qualitative and quantitative research, examined real incidences of fetal and infant death in the county, disseminated research findings through a formal report and presentation, and suggested four major implications for health professionals in Cincinnati. Unlike more traditional psychology capstone experiences in which student work does not leave the classroom environment, students in the CHD-partnered service learning capstone had the opportunity to translate research findings into meaningful deliverables that directly benefit public health in our area. The CHD also benefited from the FIMR project by gaining important insight into some of the driving mechanisms behind infant mortality. Rigorous data analysis of rich content derived directly through structured interviews with women experiencing loss provided suggestions for policy based on evidence. Because public professionals are charged with huge responsibility in delivering programming, they often do not have the time or resources to delve into the mass of available data. Through the partnership, service-learning students fill that need by devoting time to analyzing existing data. Essentially, both academic and community partners benefited through this project, and since both partners were similarly aligned based on education, research interests, student investment, and community outcomes, the partnership continued.

Project #2: Reproductive Health and Wellness Program (RHWP)

Based on the success of the FIMR project and the mutual benefits for students and the CHD, both partners identified another issue to assess in the upcoming semester. In the second project, students worked with data from the RHWP to evaluate a school-based reproductive health program for adolescents. The CHD-funded program utilizes a Community Health Worker (CHW) to provide reproductive health education to adolescents and to help connect them to reproductive health services. The program is designed to increase the number of teens who seek reproductive health care as a means to prevent unintended pregnancy and lower STI incidence, thereby indirectly addressing the infant mortality issue in our area.

Capstone students analyzed data collected by the CHW. The teens visited the CHW in their school-based health clinic for education and consultation and when requested, the CHW connected them to a RHWP clinic to receive birth control and other reproductive services. To evaluate the program, capstone students identified three research objectives: 1) to describe adolescents utilizing the services of a Community Health Worker; 2) to explore how adolescents were connected to reproductive health education and services provided by the Community Health Worker; and 3) to explore the degree age was related to reproductive health knowledge, attitudes, and behaviors.

The RHWP project directly benefited both the public health department and the capstone student collaborators. The work completed by the capstone students was useful to the public health department because grant funding has limitations for data analysts. Until this partnership, the RHWP had no real obtainable way to measure the work the CHW was doing in the field. Findings from the students' analyses indicated that the CHW was successful in her role and more teens were accessing services, thereby preventing pregnancy and STIs. The RHWP project directly benefited students by providing them with the opportunity to experience the "real life" implications for research, statistics, and report writing. This project has continued with the next semester of college students to allow for an analysis of a larger sample size and more longitudinal data.

Discussion

Over the course of eighteen months, the inter-professional collaboration between the University of Cincinnati and the Cincinnati Health Department has had three major impacts. First, academic partners integrated teaching, research, and service roles for community impact. Second, CHD has received much-needed assistance from outside researchers, uniquely able to apply scientific rigor to existing public health data. Third, the collaborative results have benefited infant vitality both directly and indirectly through addressing unintended pregnancy and other indicators of infant death. Each impact will be discussed and limitations and future directions of our long-term university-public health department partnership will be addressed.

The academic partners in our collaboration technically include both a research-track professor at a large urban university and the students enrolled in her capstone course over eighteen months. The academic partner continues to benefit significantly from the professional relationship formed with the public health partner. This academic-public health partnership provides a unique strategy to meet the research, teaching, and service requirements of academia while also making an impact in local communities. By focusing an undergraduate course on infant mortality, a topic relevant to personal research interests, the efforts of the academic professor fulfilled both research and teaching agendas. In addition, the results of the collaborative projects were directly translated to the local public health community in the form of presentations and reports, thereby contributing to community action efforts and fulfilling service requirements as well.

Students also served as academic partners in our interdisciplinary collaboration. By participating in service-learning at the health department, students had the opportunity to contribute to program enhancements through utilization of the scientific method to interpret meaningful results. Both in-class performance and feedback from students suggests that applying research methods to actual health problems in our local area enhances learning outcomes. Anecdotally, we have noticed that students become more engaged in even mundane research tasks when their purpose is important for the large goal. For example, students participating in the FIMR project carefully read countless pages of interview transcripts line-by-line to conduct qualitative analysis, staying after class and making additional time to ensure the analyses were thorough and complete. In end-of-semester course evaluations, students commonly describe the service-learning projects as highly beneficial and even transformative. Example student qualitative comments include, "I learned so much about the research process, more than any class I had taken before" and "having the opportunity to partake in research that yielded positive results for Cincinnati adolescents was the best and most rewarding thing I've ever done in any of my undergraduate classes."

The public health department in our partnership also experiences tangible benefits from the interdisciplinary collaboration. Public health departments by design are inviting to research dollars but often lack the infrastructure to manage research projects, interpret findings, and implement changes within the public health system. Service grants are sought instead since governmental positions can be posted, hired, and trained to implement the program with the grant dollars. With this, the pressure to implement a program, meet benchmarks, and apply for additional grants limits the capabilities of finding influential relationships in data. Therefore, much of the service provision grants cannot be rooted in real evidence because it has yet to be discovered. Public health departments are minefields for data but few have the skills and time to run analysis and interpret findings. Collaboration between both partners led to enhancing the FIMR and RHWP programs by increasing rigorous data analysis, and demonstrating efficacy in program expansion, respectively.

In addition to impact on academic and public health partners, the inter-professional collaboration also had direct and indirect impacts on infant vitality in our area. CHD's goal of eliminating health disparities and promoting health equity are better actualized with interdisciplinary collaboration since individual bias can be reduced, diversity is invited, and resources are pooled. By reducing unintended pregnancy in our region and by understanding the social forces behind infant loss, the two projects our partnership has completed will help promote the health and well being of young women, infants, and families. Evidence-based programs promote our community by increasing opportunities to improve socioeconomic conditions and the career aptitude of the community. The care of undeserved women and men is an area of focus all its own and involves knowledge of the social determinants of health inequity and systematic approach to improving outcomes.

Prior to the academic-public health department collaboration there have been no scientific evaluations of the quality of these programs. Without evaluation, program development and improvement would be arbitrary. Data obtained from the two projects described is crucial for the improvement of programs aimed at reducing infant mortality. Consistent with the work of existing collaborations, this partnership utilized the principles of successful collaboration – common interests and goals, mutual cooperation and shared responsibility, and expected mutual benefit (13). In addition, this partnership found a way to be sustainable through replication. Each semester, the partnership renews and the principles are carefully reassessed prior to implementation.

In addition to the significant benefits experienced through our university-public health department partnership, we have dealt with challenges along the way. Many obstacles come in the form of logistical challenges that take some additional planning and compromise to overcome. For example, students enrolled in the capstone course often lack flexibility in their schedules, so activities with the health department are essentially limited to class time. Meetings at the health department are limited to no more than one hour to allow students to travel back to campus to attend classes immediately following ours. As principal collaborators, our project planning is limited to activities that do not require student attendance outside class time. Similarly, each project is limited to that which can be completed during the 10 weeks of an academic semester.

Some challenges also fell on the public health side of the partnership. For the RHWP project, we have overcome the semester challenge by designing the course to build on the results from the previous semester. Challenges from the public health side include issues with data cleaning and confidentiality. All data must be coded and cleaned prior to student analysis. This took additional time for the public health partner to complete so that informative results could be derived. In addition, data had to be de-identified according to the confidentiality standards set by the Department of Health and Human Services (HHA). Finally, as a former professor in the academic setting the public health partner was enthusiastic about teaching a few class sessions each semester, although lecture preparation took place outside the normal work day.

In conclusion, an academic-public health department collaboration that partners with psychology undergraduates to investigate locally relevant public health phenomena can be an effective strategy to meet both academic and public health department goals. By committing to a long-term partnership rather than single projects, the collaboration is better able to address the larger public health issue of infant mortality.

References

[1] Jacquez F, Mooney J. Identifying themes in Fetal and Infant Mortality Review (FIMR) interviews. Cincinnati, OH: Department of Psychology, University of Cincinnati, 2012.

[2] James M Anderson Center for Health Systems Excellence. Preventing infant mortality. URL: http://www.cincinnatichildrens.org/service/j/anderson-center/community-population-health/infant-mortality/

[3] Larkin M, Richardson E, Tabreman J. New partnerships in health and social care for an era of public spending cuts. Health Soc Care Commun 2011;20(2):199-207.

[4] Wehrens R, Bekker M, Bal R. Coordination of research, policy and practice: A case study of collaboration in the field of public health. Sci Public Policy 2011;38(10):755-66.

[5] Pistella CY, Synkewecz CA. Community postpartum care needs assessment and systems development for low income families. J Health Soc Policy 1999;11(1):53-64.

[6] Gipson JD, Koenig MA, Hindin MJ. The effects of unintended pregnancy on infant, child, and parental health: A review of the literature. Stud Fam Plann 2008;39(1):18-38.

[7] The Guttmacher Institute. Family planning can reduce high infant mortality levels. New York, 2002. URL: http://www.guttmacher.org/pubs/ib_2-02.pdf

[8] D'Angelo DV, Gilbert BC, Rochat RW, Santelli JS, Herold JM. Differences between mistimed and unwanted pregnancies among women who have live births. Perspect Sex Reprod H 2002;36(5):192-7.

[9] Orr ST, Reiter JP, James SA, Orr CA. Maternal health prior to pregnancy and preterm birth among urban, low income black women in Baltimore: The Baltimore preterm birth study. Ethn Dis 2011;22(1):85-9.

[10] Shanok AF, Miller L. Depression and treatment with inner city pregnant and parenting teens. Arch Womens Ment Health 2007;10(5):199-210.

[11] Patel PH, Sen B. Teen motherhood and long-term health consequences. Matern Child Health J 2012;16:1063-71.

[12] Sullivan BA. Inter-organizatonal relationships of health partnerships: Characteristics of the Fulton County Sparc Program. J Health Hum Serv Adm 2012;35(1):44-70.

[13] Staton-Tindall M, Rees JD, Oser CB, McNees B, Mooney Palmer J. Establishing partnerships between correctional agencies and university researchers to enhance substance abuse treatment initiatives. Corrections Today 2007:42-45.

[14] Petroro R, Marola M, Ferreira T, Raboin K, Lewis KK. A win-win partnership between academia and public health practice. Public Health Nurs 2011;28(6):543-7.

[15] Landry L, Lee R, Greenwald J. The San Francisco collaborative: An evaluation of a partnership between three schools of nursing and a public health department. Public Health Nurs 2011;26(6):568-73.

[16] Johnston SC, Hauser SL, Desmond-Hellmann S. Enhancing ties between academia and industry to improve health. Nature Med 2011;17(4):434-6.

[17] Taylor-Robinson DC, Loyd-Williams F, Orton L, Moonan M, O'Flaherty M, Capewell S. Barriers to partnership working in public health: A qualitative study. PLoS ONE 2012;7(1): 1-8.

[18] Maseru N. Cincinnati Health Department Mission Statement. Cincinnati Health Department, Cincinnati, OH, United States of America. URL: http://www.cincinnati-oh.gov/health/

Section three: Inter-professional community work

In: Public Health
Editors: Rosemary M. Caron and Joav Merrick

ISBN: 978-1-63321-569-6

Chapter 11

Community wise: A group behavioral intervention

Liliane Cambraia Windsor*, PhD, MSW[1], Lauren Jessell, LSW[1], Teri Lassiter, PhD[2] and Ellen Benoit, PhD[3]

[1]School of Social Work and [2]School of Public Health, Rutgers The State University of New Jersey, Newark, New Jersey and [3]National Development and Research Institutes, New York, US

Individuals with histories of incarceration and substance abuse residing in distressed communities often receive suboptimal services partly due to a lack of empirically supported substance abuse treatments targeting this population. Grounded in community-engaged research, we developed *Community Wise*, a manualized, 12-week, group behavioral intervention. The intervention aims to reduce substance use frequency, HIV/HCV risk behaviors, and reoffending among individuals with histories of substance abuse and incarceration. Thirty-six individuals were recruited to participate in a formative evaluation of *Community Wise* processes and outcomes. Analysis showed significantly lower post-intervention number of cigarettes smoked per day, days using an illicit drug, money spent on illegal drugs, and rearrests. Based on the evaluation, the research team made the following changes: 1) added a session on sexuality; 2) increased the number of sessions from 12 to 15; and 3) modified strategies to help participants develop and implement capacity building projects.

Introduction

Health disparities in the United States are well documented and result in a significant financial burden to the nation. For example, the per capita rate of new AIDS cases is 9.4 times higher for Blacks than it is for Whites (1). These differences, as identified by the National Healthcare Disparities Report, mandated by Congress, impose great financial and human costs. According to the Joint Center for Political and Economic Studies, health disparities cost

* Correspondence: Liliane Cambraia Windsor, PhD, MSW, 360 Martin Luther King Jr. Blvd, Hill Hall, Room 401C, Newark, NJ 07104, United States. E-mail: lwindsor@ssw.rutgers.edu.

the United States $1.24 trillion between 2003 and 2006 and this burden has only continued to grow (2). Disparities related to race and income are exacerbated in low-income African-American communities, where substance abuse and incarceration rates are high. Health indicators show that African-Americans suffer significantly harsher consequences of substance use than their White counterparts (e.g. higher rates of HIV/HCV infection), and yet, have less access to HIV and substance abuse interventions that could mitigate this disparity (3,4).

For low-income African-Americans involved in the criminal justice system, incarceration has a significant impact on health and substance use, especially upon release. Few individuals receive substance abuse treatment and HIV/HCV prevention services while in prison and they often return to the same distressed communities in which they obtained and used drugs, engaged in related risk behaviors, and became exposed to the criminal justice system (5). Research has identified this issue as a major obstacle in maintaining recovery (6,7).

Despite increased efforts to reduce health disparities in distressed African American communities, few evidence-based interventions have been successfully adopted by these communities (8). Often substance abuse and community reentry programs focus solely on individual treatment even though community-based models have been shown to enhance effectiveness by addressing the environmental context in which problems occur (9). This chapter reports results of the formative evaluation of *Community Wise,* a community-based, manualized, multilevel health intervention designed to reduce substance use frequency, HIV/HCV risk behaviors, and reoffending among individuals with histories of substance abuse and incarceration residing in distressed communities in Newark, New Jersey. The long term goal of *Community Wise* is to reduce health disparities. Distressed communities are defined as geographic areas where rates of poverty, drug use and traffic, violence, and disease are higher than in neighboring areas (10).

Developing "Community wise"

Community Based Participatory Research (CBPR) principles were used to develop and pilot-test *Community Wise*. CBPR requires that researchers and community members work together to identify community problems and solutions through the combination of scientific and experiential knowledge. The key purpose of CBPR is to help create knowledge that can be immediately used to help the community involved in the research (11,12).

Community Wise was developed by a team of community members, consumers (individuals with histories of incarceration and substance abuse and their families and friends), service providers, researchers, and government officials who compose the Newark Community Collaborative Board (NCCB). The NCCB has been working together using a CBPR framework since September 2010 to develop *Community Wise*. During phase 1 of the formative evaluation, the NCCB was formed, trained, and engaged in CBPR to conduct a needs assessment as well as an ethnographic study that informed the development of *Community Wise*. The NCCB also developed the first edition of the *Community Wise* manual (13–15). During phase 2 of the formative evaluation, *Community Wise* was implemented for the first time in the Spring of 2012 with 26 individuals at a community based agency to test the feasibility of the manual and develop the first evaluation procedures (16). The current chapter reports findings from phase 3 of the formative evaluation, where the NCCB implemented the revised version of *Community Wise*'s manual with 36 individuals at a community-based agency in Newark, NJ. Phase 3 aimed to examine the feasibility of the revised manual and maximize its potential efficacy. This paper discusses, in detail, the process implemented by the NCCB to evaluate the intervention's feasibility and the lessons learned in this process.

Theoretical framework

Community Wise was informed by Paulo Freire's critical consciousness theory (17). Freire defined critical consciousness as the ability to "perceive social, political, and economic contradictions, and to take action against the oppressive elements of reality" (p. 19). Based on this theory, vulnerable populations should be encouraged to engage in critical dialogue about the oppressive elements in their lives and communities. Critical consciousness can empower these individuals to engage in social action (e.g. engage in their communities' political process) to combat the oppression they experience (e.g. lack of access to affordable and healthy food, meaningful employment, and quality health care). Oppression can be internalized, contributing to criminal activity, substance use and other risk behaviors. Using critical consciousness theory, *Community Wise* seeks to redirect the effects of oppression away from destructive, health-risk behavior into outward, positive action such as planting a community garden and/or advocating for community resources. In order to achieve this goal, the 12 group sessions that make up *Community Wise* encourage participants to think critically and engage in dialogue about the oppression they experience. At the same time, participants are encouraged to combat oppression by working with one another to create a community capacity building project and develop the skills they need (e.g. leadership) to bring about change in their community (e.g. increasing access to quality foods) (18). Table 1 displays a summary of the intervention's sessions with respective goals.

Our project

A mixed-methods research design informed by CBPR was implemented to test *Community Wise's* feasibility. Quantitative methods consisted of process measures and a pre-posttest design to gauge changes in substance use frequency, HIV/HCV risk behaviors, and reoffending before and after the intervention. Qualitative methods consisted of analyzing four focus groups with *Community Wise* participants to explore participants' feedback about the intervention and qualitative analysis of session video digital recordings to explore the development of critical consciousness and the application of *Community Wise's* key ingredients. The findings were then combined to inform revisions made to the manual and the research protocol. The current chapter will focus on the qualitative component of the evaluation as the quantitative component is being covered in more detail elsewhere (19).

Table 1. Intervention sessions and respective goals

Session # and Theme	Overall Goals
Session 1: Icebreaker and Welcome	*To introduce participants and facilitators to one another, To present an overview of Community Wise To establish ground rules*
Session 2: Critical Thinking	*To explore critical thinking literature and evaluate one's own thinking patterns*
Session 3: Solar System	*To use the solar system as a metaphor to help participants explore power dynamics and the role of community building and civic engagement as empowerment tools*
Session 4: Empowerment	*To help participants development personal goals and a capacity building project as empowerment strategies*
Session 5: Funhouse Mirrors	*To use the funhouse mirrors metaphor to help participants explore the impact of internalized and structural oppression on their communities, thinking patterns, and risk behaviors*
Session 6: Empowerment	*To help participant develop personal goals and a capacity building project as empowerment strategies*
Session 7: Walls	*To use the metaphor of confining walls to help participants identify oppressive structural systems and appropriate strategies for overcoming them*
Session 8: Empowerment	*To provide support to participants as they attempt to implement their personal goals and capacity building projects*
Session 9: Historical Trauma	*To examine the impact of historical trauma on participants' present behaviors*
Session 10: Empowerment	*To support participants in evaluating progress and addressing challenges in their personal goals and capacity building projects*
Session11: Family structure and dynamics	*To explore how different family structures and dynamics may influence both positively and negatively the perpetuation of structural and internalized oppression*
Session 12: Termination and Personal Evaluation	*To help participants work through feelings that arise from ending group work and to articulate orally new skills and ways of thinking acquired through their participation in Community Wise. Participants are encouraged to share how new skills and ways of thinking may help them accomplish longer term plans*
Graduation	*Participants celebrate their work, and engage with community members to raise awareness about substance abuse, HIV/ HCV risk behaviors, and reoffending*

Staff and NCCB training and monitoring

The current evaluation was conducted after obtaining approval from the Institutional Review Board (IRB) at two partner universities and at the community based organization where groups were held. Social workers and research support staff were directly supervised by the Principal Investigator (PI). The staff received training on study measures, data collection, and the *Community Wise* manual. Members of the NCCB received training on CBPR principles and philosophy, ethical treatment of research participants, and research methods and procedures. NCCB members met monthly to review and approve research procedures, resolve any challenges, and make decisions about potential changes to the manual and the research protocol.

Sample recruitment

Participants were recruited by the NCCB using purposive sampling. Specifically, recruitment flyers were distributed to service providers and potential study participants who contacted the study's phone number so that people could help spread the information to friends, family members, and acquaintances. To be eligible, participants had to have been incarcerated within the past four years, have a history of substance abuse within the past year, be 18 years of age or older, reside in Essex County, NJ, speak English and provide informed consent. Participants were screened by a masters-level social worker using standardized measures (20–23). Participants were deemed ineligible if they were found to have a high level of suicidality, an unstabilized psychotic disorder, gross cognitive impairment or did not have a moderate to high level of drug and/or alcohol use in the past year.

Participants received $15 for completing a clinical screening. Individuals who met eligibility criteria were invited to participate in *Community Wise* and distributed into four intervention groups based on gender and availability. Study staff reviewed a written consent form, outlining the risks and benefits of participating and a certificate of confidentiality obtained from the federal government to prohibit court-ordered violations of participants' confidentiality. In signing the consent form, participants agreed to have all *Community Wise* sessions video-taped and to use code names during the group sessions to protect their confidentiality. Seventy-nine participants completed a phone screening followed by a clinical screening to assess eligibility. Forty individuals were assigned to *Community Wise* and 36 completed the 12-week data collection follow-up.

Procedures

The qualitative evaluation included four focus groups (one focus group for each *Community Wise* group) which occurred after the *Community Wise* sessions were completed. The purpose of the focus groups was to obtain feedback from participants. An NCCB member and a research assistant hired specifically to fulfill this role conducted the focus groups. All 40 participants who attended at least one *Community Wise* session were invited to participate. Those who participated received $20.

Group facilitators attended weekly clinical supervision with the project PI. Clinical supervision ensured treatment fidelity and provided facilitators with feedback. During supervision, the group discussed challenges, ensured that the manual was being implemented accurately, and discussed non-responsive clients. The PI watched all session videos and completed a checklist to provide feedback to facilitators.

Data analysis

Data from qualitative analyses included a random sample of 23 out of 48 digital videos of group sessions and verbatim transcriptions of focus groups. The focus group transcripts were coded and analyzed manually by one of the authors and a thematic analysis was conducted (24). This process involves reading the data several times, coding and recoding through a process of constant comparison until themes and categories become clear. The focus group data complemented quantitative measures of participant feedback. Such triangulation helps ensure completeness of data and can reveal convergence or dissonance in key themes developed in our analyses (25).

Video data was open coded by two research assistants using N-vivo qualitative data analysis software. Inter-rater reliability was calculated reaching over 90% agreement on all codes. The codes were then analyzed for common themes by the PI and two NCCB members. The research questions included: 1) What were the main *Community Wise* ingredients impacting critical consciousness, drug use frequency, HIV/HCV risk behaviors, and reoffending?; and 2) Were these ingredients successfully implemented and if not, how should they be modified?

Findings

A total of 36 individuals participated in this study. Ninety-four percent were African-American; most were heterosexual, single, unemployed and reported a mean household yearly income of less than $10,000. Most were not currently supervised by the criminal justice system. The charge associated with participant's last incarceration varied; the most common charges were drug possession, property and technical violations, and violent crimes. On average, participants had been released from their last incarceration 13 months prior to the intervention. All participants were either using an illicit drug or alcohol at the time of baseline or reported use within the past year. Most were smoking an average of ten cigarettes per day at the time of baseline. Ten percent reported being HIV positive and 11% reported being HCV positive. Table 1 displays the sample's demographic characteristics. Table 2 displays participants' demographics.

Intervention retention

Participants completed an average of 7 (± 3.85) out of 12 sessions. Participants were defined as having successfully completed the intervention if they attended six or more group sessions and showed clinical improvement. Clinical improvement was established in clinical supervision and measured by specific progress that each participant made on personal goals, participation in capacity building projects, and improvement on distal outcomes. Seventy percent successfully completed the intervention. Completion was defined based on previous work examining other behavioral interventions in the literature (26,27). Specifically, successful completion included those who attended at least 7 sessions, demonstrated clinical improvement (e.g.: reduced drug use, improved mental health symptoms), and engaged in capacity building projects.

Table 2. Participants' characteristics at baseline (N=36)

Characteristic	N (%) or Mean (±SD)
Male	18 (49)
Heterosexual	32 (89)
Age	44.65 (±8.4)
Race	
Black/African American	34 (94)
White	2 (06)
Ethnicity	
Hispanic	3 (07)
Not Hispanic	33 (93)
Household yearly income	7,340.73 (±9,805.5)
Religion	
Christian	24 (67)
Muslim/Islam	8 (22)
None	4 (11)
Marital Status	
Single/never married	18 (57)
Unemployed	33 (91)
Criminal Justice System Status	
Parole	4 (10)
Probation	5 (13)
No supervision	27 (77)
Number of months since release from incarceration	13 (±13.8)
Criminal Charge at Last Incarceration	
Violent crime (assault, homicide, carjacking, robbery)	4 (12)
Property crime (burglary, fraud, shoplifting)	13 (36)
Drug Possession	13 (36)
Drug dealing	1 (02)
Sex Work	1 (02)
Warrants/technical violations	4 (12)
Reporting committing any crime(s) above since last incarceration	8 (22)
Substance Use	% (n) or mean (±SD)
Any alcohol use past 30 days	38 (±61)
Number of heavy drinking days (past 90-days)	25.5 (±32.8)
Average Drinks per drinking day (past 90-days)	10.2 (±20.0)
Number of Current Smokers	55 (±89)
Number of Cigarettes per day	10.5 (±10.3)
Reported illicit drug use past 90 days (cocaine/opiates/marijuana)	13 (±79)
Number of days any illicit drug use past 90 days (cocaine/opiates/marijuana)	33.9 (±32.7)
Money spent on illicit drug per using day	41.4 (±30.2)
Testing positive for drug use	22 (60)

Table 2. (Continued)

Characteristic	N (%) or Mean (±SD)
HIV/HCV Status and HIV/HCV Risk/Protective Factors	
HIV + HCV+	4 (10) 5 (11)
Average number of times tested for HIV Average number of times tested for HCV	7.5 (±9.9) 5.0 (±8.7)
Number of times engaging in risky drug use in past 30 days	0.9 (±5.1)
Frequency of engagement in risky sexual behaviors	0.5 (±0.3)*
Psychological Distress**	
PTSD*** (responding yes to having had a near death experience)	20 (57)
PTSQ (PTSD Symptom Severity)	1.1 (±0.7)
BSI 18 Total Score	0.7 (±0.7)
Attitudes Toward Research Average # agreeing that research is important Average # agreeing that research procedures were easy to understand Average # agreeing that researchers do not always inform participants about the risks involved in health research	31 (87) 21 (59) 13 (37)

* Indicates that in average participants reported either never engaging or only engaging a few times in sex risk behaviors.
**Ranges from 0 to 4 (higher scores mean higher psychological distress).
***Ranges from 0 to 3 (higher scores mean higher PTSD symptom severity).

Findings from focus groups

A total of 25 out of 40 participants attended the focus groups. Analysis revealed two overall themes: 1) Participant satisfaction with the intervention, and 2) Areas of strengths and areas that need to be improved. Overall, focus group participants reported that the intervention was useful, with many expressing a desire to maintain contact with the program post-graduation as a means of continuing their personal growth and development. Participants identified group facilitators and the participant's manual as key factors in their satisfaction with C*ommunity Wise*. According to participants, the facilitators were viewed as a source of knowledge and information, as well as providing a support mechanism for some of the participants. For instance, a male participant noted that his facilitator took time from his schedule to check on him when he had no one else to turn to, which in turn provided the motivation he needed to continue the program. Participants reported the manual was useful in helping them think about the group work outside of group and it was a way to share what they were learning with others.

Participants had a few suggestions to improve the intervention. A female participant believed it was unrealistic to complete a capacity building project in twelve weeks. One of the male participants agreed and in order to address this issue in his group, they decided to meet outside of the scheduled sessions, at a participant's home, to "carry on our part of our project that we still feel we want to see through to the end." Finally, participants felt that *Community*

Wise should provide them with concrete job leads and references to increase their chances of gainful employment; according to them, this should be the first priority of the intervention.

Findings from session videos

Analysis revealed Community Wise's mechanisms of change which included two overall domains: 1) Operational ingredients; and 2) Active ingredients. Figure 1 displays the mechanisms of change.

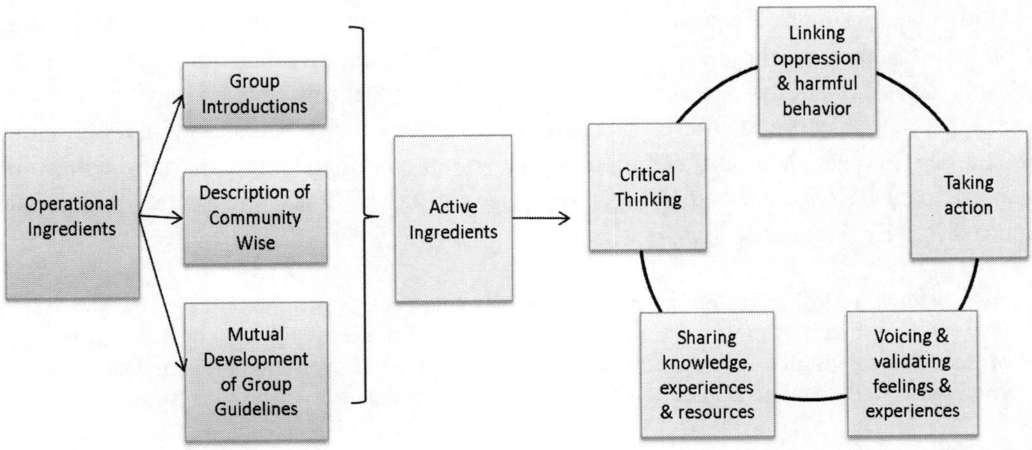

Figure 1. Community Wise's Mechanisms of Change.

Operational ingredients are intended to create a safe environment where the intervention can thrive. These included group introductions, a description of *Community Wise*'s background, and the mutual development of group guidelines. Combined, these activities served as a way for the facilitator to establish confidence, trust and commitment among the group members. For instance, in establishing group norms and expectations, the facilitators explained *Community Wise's* background to the participants, how the intervention was developed, and their personal commitment to it. Group norms and expectations were established by the participants themselves, who were encouraged during the beginning few sessions to come up with their own group guidelines. The guidelines were revisited throughout the intervention, as expectations changed and commitment to the group grew.

The active ingredients of Community Wise comprised activities that seemed to impact the development of critical consciousness and distal outcomes. These activities included 1) critical thinking; 2) identifying and discussing the link between oppression and harmful behavior; 3) taking action; 4) voicing & validating each other's feelings and experiences; and 5) sharing knowledge, experiences, and resources. Figure 1 displays *Community Wise's* mechanisms of change.

Critical thinking involved the group participants questioning information and examining the quality of their own thinking process, often as a result of the homework assignments (e.g. reading an article about Crack Baby syndrome or researching and questioning HIV conspiracy theories) and the group dialogue. In thinking critically, participants linked structural oppression to their behavior and means of coping. For example, in the women's group, participants discussed the article about crack baby syndrome and whether or not it is a real problem or just a myth. Before reading the article, the group shared their experiential knowledge about this topic, with many women describing the sick babies they met in their lives. Then, they read the article and posed critical questions (e.g.: How do you know what you know is true? What information is more reliable: Scientific? Experiential? Coming from authorities?). The discussion finally culminated with the question: What are the consequences if I believe that the crack baby syndrome is true? And what are the consequences if I believe it is not true? The group engaged in a deep discussion about the role of racism, stigma, and classism in the production of knowledge and how these macro level issues impact their individual beliefs and behaviors.

Understanding and identifying the role of oppression was stressed by the group facilitators throughout the sessions. The homework, exercises and prompts from the facilitators and one another encouraged participants to connect the role of oppression to the choices that they make in relation to substance use, HIV/HCV risk behavior, and reoffending. For example, in reacting to an illustration of a person of color engaging in harmful behaviors, one participant described how the negative image he has of himself in society makes him want to drink. He explained,

> "…to keep certain images out of my mind and by the time they added all up you know, they may not be all of them mirrors but there's a couple of them mirrors, not really proud of it, and in my mind it's like well don't think about that and my weakness was just, well you won't really have to think about it if you just have a few more drinks, you know?"

Taking action is another active ingredient that seemed to impact critical consciousness and distal outcomes among participants. Throughout the group sessions, participants were encouraged to respond to their experiences of structural oppression by taking action against it. They were encouraged to do this by setting and talking about personal goals and by organizing a capacity building project amongst themselves. For example, one of the participants described how no matter how hard he tries he can't find employment: "I filled out 1,000 applications, no exaggeration…" The participants in this group eventually agreed to create a community garden where they would grow vegetables and sell them in a farmers market. In taking action, this participant started to respond to the oppression in his life by supporting his community. Rather than harming himself, he was encouraged to work with other participants to react in a more positive and action-oriented way, creating his own employment opportunity.

Voicing and validating each other's experiences and anger related to structural oppression was another active ingredient of *Community Wise*. It allowed participants to give and receive support and to articulate experiences related to oppression that are not always acknowledged. Participants described the frustration they faced trying to achieve financial stability and shelter while having a criminal history. One participant talked about his steps to join a protest group in Newark, NJ representing the unemployed and another discussed getting denied low-income housing because they don't accept ex-offenders:

> "I'm just like yesterday and today I just been like real frustrated you know because like I'm trying to do what I can to you know better myself and it's like I keep hitting brick walls…"

This participant then went on to say that he can't allow himself to act on his frustration by returning to illegal activities because that will just lead him back to "prisons, institutions and death." Issues related to structural oppression were also discussed from the homework assignments and activities and again, participants received validation and the freedom to express their anger in a supportive environment. In providing one another with a means to express their anger and hardships, they were able to engage in critical dialogue to develop community engaged ways to combat the oppression they were facing.

Sharing knowledge, experiences and resources served as an additional way of responding to oppression, this time by empowering one another and exchanging information. Perhaps as a result of talking about the oppression in their lives and supporting each other throughout the group sessions, participants began working together to share resources and knowledge they had about jobs, social service benefits, housing options and other useful resources with one another. They also began using one another as resources, supporting each other through the challenges they went through during the week. As the weeks went on, participants worked together as a team, not just on the capacity building projects but also to support one another individually to make better choices related to their health and behavior. For example, participants encouraged each other to avoid substance abuse and other harmful behavior, asking that they call other group members before engaging in risky behavior, rather than after. One participant in the women's group talked about how she has been thinking about calling the co-facilitator who attends 12-step meetings and that she was contemplating going back to meetings and "getting clean" again:

> "I know meetings work for me, they kept me clean for multiple years, over a decade. So I know that but I dunno, I just know I've got new hope with going back to work and getting a pay check like I used to get before I got fired I got a pay check so I've got a little renewed hope."

In getting her basic needs met (e.g. obtaining a job), this participant expressed being more motivated to stop using substances. The group encouraged this participant to reach out to them and to use resources in the community, such as a detox center and 12-step meetings.

While the ingredients appeared to work and affect change in two of the groups, they did not work as well in the third. This may have been due to the facilitator's failure to establish a belief in the group's ability, such as their capacity to create and follow group guidelines. Also, critical thinking was not explained well by this facilitator as a means to recognize oppression and the link between oppression and harmful behavior was not well established. These issues may have had a negative impact on the ingredients' ability to affect change among the participants in this group.

Discussion

Findings from this process evaluation showed that *Community Wise* was acceptable to individuals with a history of substance abuse and incarceration residing in a distressed community. Participants found the intervention useful and process measures revealed strong alliance and a high retention rate in the intervention, considering this is such a hard to reach and hard to engage population (19,28). Overall, the results suggest that participants were able to engage in treatment and viewed the intervention as beneficial, despite the multiple challenges they face (e.g. homelessness, unemployment, poverty).

Analysis of process measures indicated a high level of satisfaction with *Community Wise* through high scores in working alliance and group climate. Participants reported finding the intervention useful and reported intent to use the skills they learned in the *Community Wise* groups (19). *Community Wise* retention rates were higher than retention rates reported in the literature from evidence-based substance abuse treatment evaluations with substance abusing individuals. Specifically, 70% of *Community Wise's* participants successfully completed treatment. Literature reporting findings from cognitive behavioral therapy evaluations with this population reveal an average of only 58% completion rates (29,30).

The mechanisms of change identified in the qualitative analysis indicated key operational and active ingredients that, when implemented by the facilitator according to the *Community Wise* manual, seemed to affect change among the participants. Some of these activities, however, were not implemented as well as they could have been. For example, the facilitator in the third group did not implement the group introductions, critical thinking or group guidelines activities as indicated in the manual. Other problems with activities consisted of issues with the intervention itself. The NCCB worked together to modify *Community Wise* in order to resolve these issues.

For example, the "taking action" mechanism of change activity of engaging in capacity building projects still needed further development. Participants encountered challenges when developing and implementing the capacity building projects, likely causing frustration, and it was difficult to measure the impact of these projects on the community. Initially, the capacity building projects were designed to be individual projects. Approximately 3 weeks into the intervention, we realized that these should be group projects for several reasons: First, critical consciousness is developed through dialogue and group work. The focus must be on process and on the skills that are learned and developed collectively by the groups. Thus, we changed the rules midway and allowed the groups to develop group projects. The next challenge happened when participants started to develop very large ideas and struggled to break them down into small, accomplishable steps. By the time the groups were finally able to agree on a small and feasible project, the groups were ending. The capacity building projects are supposed to help participants learn group working skills, connect with others in their communities, and feel proud of the community work they accomplish. In this formative evaluation however, only one group was able to implement their capacity building project.

In addition to problems with the capacity building projects, qualitative analysis of video sessions indicated a lack of content specific to sexuality issues and challenges with the design of capacity building projects. It is likely that these weaknesses in the manual are at least partially responsible for the lack of significant changes in HIV/HCV risk behavior (see the Lessons Learned/ Manual Changes section below). Due to methodological limitations (e.g.: lack of a control group), it is not possible to conclude that the intervention caused the changes in outcomes (19). However, pre- to post-intervention changes in outcome measures seem to indicate that *Community Wise* has the potential to be helpful as indicated by many favorable outcome changes in the expected direction. Small to large positive effect sizes were found for the overall sample in all of the outcomes. Findings were especially promising for substance abuse and reoffending outcomes as many of these variables reached statistical significance despite the small sample. However, no statistically significant changes were found in

HIV/HCV risk behaviors (19). These findings replicate results from *Community Wise's* cohort 1(16).

Lessons learned/manual changes

Once the process evaluation data analysis was completed, findings were presented to the NCCB and discussed to determine implications and future steps. The NCCB agreed to meet for a retreat in which changes to the manual, guided by the research findings and by the NCCB's experiential knowledge, would be discussed and implemented. The NCCB agreed to increase the number of sessions from 12 to 15, with two of the additional sessions dedicated to discussions about the capacity building projects and one session focused on sexuality. The goal of the sexuality session will be to explore homophobia and sexism as forms of oppression and to understand the impact of this oppression on behavioral health and HIV/HCV risk behaviors.

The NCCB also spent a great deal of time discussing the capacity building projects. Members agreed that capacity building projects must focus on process, rather than project outcomes, with step by step guidelines on how to best research and implement goals. The projects must be feasible and accomplishable in a short period of time. We are currently developing the model that participants will follow as they engage in their capacity building projects.

Conclusion

While data provides evidence indicating that *Community Wise* is a promising intervention, formative evaluation indicates that future development and research is needed to test the mechanisms of change and the real effect of *Community Wise* on distal and proximal outcomes. Funding is currently being sought to conduct a randomized clinical trial to test the efficacy of the revised manual of *Community Wise*.

Acknowledgments

The project described was supported by the Center for Behavioral Health Services and Criminal Justice Research (CBHSR), which is funded by the National Institute of Mental Health, award number P30MH079920 and by the HIV Intervention Science Training Program for Promising New Investigators from Underrepresented Groups (HISTP), funded by the National Institutes of Health (NIH), award number R25MH080665. The content is solely the responsibility of the authors and does not necessarily represent the official views of the National Institute of Mental Health, the National Institutes of Health, CBHS, Rutgers University, HISTP, or Columbia University. We would like to acknowledge the contributions made by all members of the Newark Community Collaborative Board and *Community Wise* participants in the development of this work.

References

[1] Centers for Disease Control. HIV among African Americans. Atlanta, GA: CDC, 2011.

[2] LaVeist TA, Gaskin DJ. The economic burden of health inequalities in the United States. Washington, DC: Joint Center for Political and Economic Studies, 2009.

[3] Warnecke RB, Oh A, Breen N, Gehlert S, Paskett E, Tucker KL, et al. Approaching health disparities from a population perspective: The National Institutes of Health Centers for Population Health and Health Disparities. Am J. Public Health 2008;98(9):1608–15.

[4] Allen K. Barriers to treatment for addicted african-american women. J Natl Med Assoc 1995;87(10):751–6.

[5] Weinbaum CM. Sabin KM, Santibanez SS. Hepatitis B, Hepatitis C, and HIV in correctional populations: A review of epidemiology and prevention. AIDS 2005;19(Suppl 3):S41–6.

[6] Shorkey C, Windsor L, Spence R. Assessing and developing cultural competence/ relevance in chemical dependence treatment organizations that serve mexican american clients and their families. J Behav Health Serv Res 2009;36(1):61–74.

[7] Windsor L, Dunlap E. What is substance use all about? Assumptions in New York's drug policies and the perceptions of drug using low-income african-americans. J Ethn Subst Abuse 2010;9(1):64–87.

[8] Schmidt L, Greenfield T, Mulia N. Unequal treatment: Racial and ethnic disparities in alcoholism treatment services. Alcohol Res Heal 2006;29(1):49–54.

[9] Trickett EJ. Multilevel community-based culturally situated interventions and community impact: an ecological perpective. Am J Commun Psychol 2009;43:257–66.

[10] Dunlap E, Golub A, Johnson BD. The severely-distressed african american family in the crack era: empowerment is not enough. J Sociol Soc Welfare 2006; 33(1):115–139.

[11] Israel B, Schultz A, Parker E, Becker A, Allen A, Guzman R. Critical issues in developing and following community based participatory research principles. In: Minkler M, Wallerstein N, Hall B, eds. Community-based participatory research for Health. San Francisco, CA: Jossey-Bass, 2008.

[12] Pinto RM, Spector AY, Valera PA. Exploring group dynamics for integrating scientific and experiential knowledge in Community Advisory Boards for HIV research. AIDS Care 2011;23(8):1006–13.

[13] Windsor L. Using concept mapping for community-based participatory research: Paving the way for community-based health interventions for oppressed populations. J Mix Methods Res 2013;7(3):274–93.

[14] Windsor L, Murugan V. From the individual to the community: Perspectives about substance abuse services. Soc Work Pract Addict 2012;12(4):412–33.

[15] Ivanova T. Due process: Breaking the cycle, 2012. Accessed 2013 Jun 05. URL: http://www.youtube.com/watch?v=0udmYxCyjw4

[16] Windsor L, Benoit E, Jemal A. Community wise: Paving the way for empowerment in community reentry. Int J Law Psychiatry, in press.

[17] Freire P. Pedagogy of the oppressed. New York: Continuum, 1976:164.

[18] Windsor L, Pinto RM, Benoit E, Jessell L, Jemal A. Community wise: Addressing oppression to promote individual and community health. Manus submitted, 2013.

[19] Windsor L, Pinto RM, Jessell L. Pilot testing Community wise: An innovative intervention to decrease health disparities. Manus submitted, 2013.

[20] Folstein M, Folstein S, McHugh P, Fanjiang G. Mini-Mental State Examination user's guide. Odessa, FL: Psychological Assessment Resources, 2001.

[21] Sheehan DV, Lecrubier Y, Harnett-Sheehan K, Amorim P, Janavs J, Weiller E, et al. The M.I.N.I. International Neuropsychiatric Interview (M.I.N.I.): The development and validation of a structured diagnostic psychiatric interview. J Clin Psychiatry 1998;59:22–33.

[22] Blanchard KA, Morgenstern J, Morgan TJ, Labouvie EW, Bux DA. Assessing consequences of substance use: Psychometric properties of the Inventory of Drug Use Consequences. Psychol Addict Behav 2003;17(4):328–31.

[23] Sobell LC, Sobell MB. Timeline followback: A technique for assessing self-reported alcohol consumption. In: Litten RZ, Allen J, eds. Measuring alcohol consumption. New Jersey: Humana Press, 1992:41–72.

[24] Braun V, Clarke V. Using thematic analysis in psychology. Qual Res Psychol 2006;3(2):77–101.

[25] Farmer T, Robinson K, Elliott SJ, Eyles J. Developing and implementing a triangulation protocol for qualitative health research. Qual Health Res 2006;16(3):377–94.

[26] Pinto RM, Campbell ANC, Hien DA, Yu G, Gorroochurn P. Retention in the National Institute on Drug Abuse Clinical Trials Network Women and Trauma Study: Implications for posttrial implementation. Am J Orthopsychiatry 2011;81(2):211–7.

[27] Windsor L, Jemal A, Alessi E. Cognitive behavioral therapy: A meta-analysis of race and substance use outcomes. Manus submitted, 2013

[28] Lewis C, Johnson BD, Golub A, Dunlap E. Studying crack abusers: Strategies for recruiting the right tail of an ill-defined population. J Psychoactive Drugs 1992;24(4):323–36.

[29] Carroll KM, Nich C, Lapaglia DM, Peters EN, Easton CJ, Petry NM. Combining cognitive behavioral therapy and contingency management to enhance their effects in treating cannabis dependence: less can be more, more or less. Addiction 2012;107(9):1650–9.

[30] Epstein DH, Hawkins WE, Covi L, Umbricht A, Preston KL. Cognitive-behavioral therapy plus contingency management for cocaine use: findings during treatment and across 12-month follow-up. Psychol Addict Behav 2003;17(1):73–82.

In: Public Health
Editors: Rosemary M. Caron and Joav Merrick
ISBN: 978-1-63321-569-6

Chapter 12

Bridge to care for refugee health

Ruth Margalit, MD*[*1], Laura Vinson, MPH[1], Christine Ngaruiya, MD[2], Kara Gehring, MPH[3], Pam Franks, BSN[4], Caci Schulte[5], Andrew Lemke, BA[5], Joshua Blood[5], Tyler Irvine, BAS[1], Chelsea Souder, BS[1], Deeko Hassan, BS[5], Andrea Langeveld, BS[6], Carolyn Corn, BS[5], Thu Hong Bui, PharmD[5] and Ann Marie Kudlacz, BSA[7]

[1]Service Learning Academy, College of Public Health, University of Nebraska Medical Center (UNMC), Omaha
[2]Department of Emergency Medicine, Yale New Haven Hospitals, New Haven, Connecticut, [3]Public Health Project Coordinator, CityMatCH, Omaha
[4]Embrace the Nations, Omaha
[5]College of Pharmacy, UNMC, Omaha, [6]College of Medicine, UNMC, Omaha
[7]Southern Sudan Community Association, Omaha, Nebraska, US

The United States resettles tens of thousands of refugees annually, with hundreds placed in mid-sized Midwestern cities such as Omaha, Nebraska. Prior to resettlement, refugees have limited access to health services and arrive with inadequate knowledge on basic hygiene practices, general healthcare issues, and minimal understanding of the American healthcare system. Additionally, current training for healthcare practitioners in the United States on issues related to refugee populations and their unique health needs are insufficient. The enormous need coupled with inadequate preparation, poses great challenges for both newly resettled refugees and health professionals, and provides opportunities for improvement with creative initiatives. The Bridge to Care (BTC) project is a unique partnership between health professions students, leaders from city and state refugee service organizations, and refugee leaders. It is a student-led/community-engaged organization overseen by the Service Learning Academy (SLA) in the College of Public

* Correspondence: Ruth Margalit MD; Associate Professor and Director, Service Learning Academy, Maurer Center for Public Health, Rm 2038; College of Public Health, Health Promotion, Social and Behavioral Health, University of Nebraska Medical Center, 986075 Nebraska Medical Center, Omaha NE 68198-4375, United States. E-mail: rmargalit@unmc.edu

Health at the University of Nebraska Medical Center. The SLA facilitates campus wide inter-professional community-based experiences like Bridge to Care. Through BTC, students take the forefront in communicating directly with leaders from community organizations and engaging with refugee leaders to determine all relevant service activities. Bridge to Care provides opportunities for students to engage in experiences that are not otherwise available in their standard curriculum. While providing essential services, students are able to enhance cultural and communication skills and gain experience working with an inter-professional team, building an understanding of the vital role each profession plays within the full spectrum of care for patients and communities.

Introduction

According to the United Nations High Commissioner for Refugees (UNHCR), a refugee is defined as someone who "owing to a well-founded fear of being persecuted for reasons of race, religion, nationality, membership of a particular social group or political opinion, is outside the country of his nationality, and is unable to, or owing to such fear, is unwilling to avail himself to the protection of that country" (1). "Secondary Migrants" are those refugees who have originally resettled in one part of the country and have subsequently moved to another location. There are approximately 15 million refugees around the world (1).

Refugees begin the process of seeking resettlement after fleeing their home countries to seek safety in neighboring nations. When refugees arrive at the nation providing asylum or temporary residence, they face three possible endpoints, one of which is resettlement in a third country such as the United States (1). This process often times takes more than 5 years while refugees live in harsh conditions within the refugee camps (1). The President of the United States sets the ceiling for refugee admission to the United States (U.S.) each fiscal year (2), for which the U.S. averages more than 50,000 refugee resettlements per year (1). Many of these refugees choose to resettle in mid-sized Midwestern cities given low costs of living and low rates of unemployment (2). Refugees are also placed in locations where existing family ties are already established (2).

Refugee resettlement in Nebraska

Currently, there are an estimated 25,000 refugees in Nebraska, with 15,000 in Omaha alone, according to Omaha resettlement agencies (personal communications) and federal resettlement reports (2, 3). In fiscal year 2013, there was a record high of 1,006 refugees resettled, and the number is expected to increase in 2014 (4). Over the years, refugees from Sudan, Somalia, Burma, Bhutan, Nepal, Iraq, Afghanistan, Ethiopia, Liberia, Congo, and Burundi have been resettled in Nebraska. As of 2006, it is estimated that over 50% of the Sudanese population in the US settled in Nebraska (5, 6). In more recent years, the majority of resettled refugees are those who have fled to camps in Thailand from nearby Burma (Myanmar) (7). The three primary refugee resettlement agencies that provide services to these refugees in Nebraska are Lutheran Family Services (LFS), Southern Sudan Community Association (SSCA), and Catholic Charities (4). The agencies provide various services such as: English classes, cultural orientation, employment assistance, fair housing education, financial literacy and household budgeting, as well as training programs for churches and civic organizations that wish to sponsor refugees and immigration legal assistance. Agencies also help coordinate access to healthcare services while in the U.S. (8).

Refugee health issues

Prior to arrival in the US, the refugee receives inadequate preparation regarding health and health-related issues (3). Refugees also lack the basic understanding about navigating the healthcare system, Western hygiene practices, preventive practices, and Western disease management (9). As a result of their circumstances, it is not unusual to find individuals with complicated health issues upon arrival and for years following resettlement. Past history of inadequate nutrition, poor sanitation, exposure to on-going violence and lack of sufficient medical care also contribute to poor health (1).

One particular area of concern is the high rates of undiagnosed infectious conditions such as tuberculosis, malaria, hepatitis C, Human Immunodeficiency Virus (HIV), as well as skin and intestinal parasites (9-11). Mental health disorders also affect a large portion of the population including a high prevalence of depression, drug and alcohol abuse (7, 11). Individuals who experienced persecution, terrorization by violent groups, imprisonment, and torture, may suffer from somatization disorders, psychosocial distress, post-traumatic stress disorder, anxiety and depression (1, 9-11). Another source of health concern is injury at the workplace (4). The majority of refugees in Omaha, Nebraska work in meat packing plants performing physically demanding jobs which puts them at high risk for injury (8).

Lastly, cultural differences distinguish America from many of the countries from which refugees originate, and these differences extend to healthcare (12). For example, in Somalia, only 2% of births take place in a health facility whereas in America, women are expected to deliver in the hospital. In addition, numerous Somali women have undergone female circumcision, which can increase the complexity of the birthing process (12).

Bridge to Care (BTC) was founded on principles of community-based participatory research (CBPR) and service-learning after identifying a gap in refugee health and healthcare needs. In addition to the language barrier, numerous refugees lack the cultural constructs to understand life in this country. Timely and appropriate healthcare acculturation is frequently unmet and much needed (9, 10). Refugees receive inadequate preparation prior to resettlement regarding fundamentals such as running a 'Western home', family roles, job distribution, the legal system, and navigating the education system (2).

The program is designed to prioritize the vast needs of the refugee populations, link refugees to existing services, and increase provider competence for cross cultural care. When working with refugees, BTC refers to health as "a state of complete physical, mental and social well-being and not merely the absence of disease or infirmity" (13). Few other programs have been designed to address refugee health issues through collaboration with community organizations.

The purpose of the work described in this chapter is to illustrate the unique partnership developed between a a health center with various health professions students, community, and refugee leaders to enhance the health of refugee in Omaha. With the number of interactions with individual refugees through BTC currently approaching 4,000 and continuing to grow, the project leaders seek to share this novel initiative with readers, sharing lessons learned and opportunities to grow. The Institutional Review Board of the University of Nebraska Medical Center approved parts of this project that involve research, such as implementation of surveys for the health education sessions.

Our project

Bridge to Care (BTC) was established in April 2010 as an inter-professional organization supported by the Service Learning Academy (SLA), College of Public Health at the University of Nebraska Medical Center (UNMC). It is a partnership involving students from the colleges of medicine, nursing, pharmacy, public health, and allied health, faculty, healthcare providers and community refugee service agencies. The goal is to facilitate positive healthcare outcomes for refugees by teaching them how to navigate the healthcare system, enhancing knowledge and cultural skills necessary for successful assimilation, and developing strong relationships with their communities.

This is achieved by: Discerning group specific health needs from each refugee community; providing health education, linkage to healthcare and services; and improving cultural awareness and knowledge regarding resettled refugees among healthcare providers.

BTC has three initiatives to accomplish this mission; monthly health education sessions, monthly mentoring sessions, and health fairs/ linkage to care events. Each of these initiatives requires collaboration with the community. Table 1 lists the partners of this project.

Table 1. Bridge to Care Partners

BTC Partners	Role
University of Nebraska Medical Center, College of Public Health, Service Learning Academy	Oversees the Bridge to Care program and assists in sustaining and expanding the program; Provides evidenced-based models of theory and community development, research methods for tracking and identifying evaluation process and outcomes
Southern Sudan Community Association (SSCA)	Resettlement Agency; Provides support and linkage to refugee community leaders
Lutheran Family Services (LFS)	Resettlement Agency; Provides support and linkage to refugee community leaders
Embrace the Nations	Faith-based organization providing cultural awareness training to Bridge to Care volunteers; Assists refugees in multiple areas of need and assists the public in better understanding and interacting with refugee populations
Omaha Public Schools, ESL Program	Partners for the mentoring program offered to refugee youth grades 5-12
Nebraska Department of Health and Human Services	Responsible for coordinating and administering the Refugee Resettlement Program on the state level

BTC Partners	Role
Alegent-Creighton Florence Clinic	State designated clinic assigned to provide initial health screenings/healthcare services to refugees; participates in annual health fair and various educational sessions, while linking refugees to long term healthcare
One World Community Health Center	Provides clinical supplies for health fairs and flu shots for multiple 'Flu Shot Clinics'
Douglas County Health Department	Provides health education resources and support
Walgreens Pharmacy	Provides clinical supplies and personnel for health fairs and flu shots for multiple 'Flu Shot Clinics'

Health education sessions

Health education sessions are developed with each refugee community (Sudanese, Somali, Burmese/Karen, and Bhutanese) for a period of three consecutive months. Health professions student leaders with respective refugee community leaders, work on building relationships, identifying health needs, planning the education opportunities in community settings and linking the refugee community to appropriate health services. Typically 15-40 participants attend each session.

Health education session topics have included pain management, hypertension, stroke, addiction, mental health, suicide prevention, immunizations, autism, healthy eating, using over the counter medications, and navigation of the U.S. healthcare system. When health needs are selected, refugee community leaders play an important role in identifying an appropriate session format (presentation by students or experts versus discussion groups), venue (faith gathering place – Church/mosque, community center, the familiar resettlement organization office), time/day for the session, recruitment of interpreters, as well as recruitment of refugee community members to attend. The health education sessions occur once every 2-4 weeks in the community.

BTC leadership recruits health professions students to participate in the sessions. The majority of students participating in health education sessions have no previous experience with refugees prior to their involvement with BTC. Hence, increasing the foundation of knowledge is important to foster appropriate interactions with and understanding of the populations being served.

As an introduction, at every health education session prior to the arrival of the refugees, student and faculty volunteers are required to participate in cultural awareness training about refugees and their health needs. The training is designed to enhance cultural sensitivity, increase knowledge and ensure that participants are better equipped to effectively interact with the refugees.

The training covers topics such as: the unique characteristics of the various refugee groups arriving in the U.S. and Omaha; the specific health needs of refugees; the importance of and tips on communicating effectively with various cultures regardless of race, ethnicity, culture or language proficiency.

Health-fairs/Linkage-to-care

In addition to health education and focused services (like flu-shots clinics for specific refugee communities), two major health fairs/linkage-to-care events are organized each year in response to the needs of the refugee community. These large events (up to 500 participants) offer a wide range of education opportunities, offering over 35 different resource booths in 2013, including information relating to proper hygiene, nutrition, immunizations, chronic disease management, and child health. Prescription and over the counter medication counseling is also available. Free preventative services like flu shots, screening for hypertension, diabetes, obesity, vision screening, fitting glasses, and dental services are also provided.

Mentoring program

In 2012, BTC expanded its engagement by adding the BTC Mentoring Program, partnering with Omaha Public School's, English as a Second Language (ESL) program for refugee students. Younger, school-aged children often find it easier to acculturate into the American lifestyle and can act as a great resource for their families.

Health professions students can become mentors following successful completion of a background check and training. Mentors are randomly assigned mentees and engage with them on selected Saturdays throughout the academic year, at least 12 times, covering topics concerning wellness and health. BTC has identified this venue as another way to improve communication with refugees. In the Fall of 2013, 352 refugee students participated with 20 health profession student mentors.

Findings

Since the inception of BTC (April 2010), over 700 students and over 4,000 refugees engaged together to address health needs.

Unlike other venues for volunteering, Bridge to Care is a relatively new model of healthcare outreach in the community. The track record, albeit short, has been consistent and positive. Different refugee groups throughout the city have benefitted from relevant education sessions and services. While progressing through their rigorous programs of excellence, students acquire skills and knowledge that will help them excel in their field. Such skills as compassionate care, cross cultural communication and multi-cultural care can impact their future patients who are likely to come from various cultural backgrounds.

These skills are best learned through experiential real-life learning, and the unique setting provided by BTC undoubtedly forges the place for the learning while facilitating potential better care for refugee populations in the future. Table 2 presents qualitative data illustrating community partners, refugees and students' perspectives.

In addition to asking refugees about relevant health topics and appropriate logistics to facilitate BTC programming, refugees are all asked to provide feedback through systematic evaluations through all three BTC programs; health education sessions, mentoring sessions, and health fairs/linkage to care events.

Table 2. Perspectives of partners in the Bridge to Care Program

	Community partner	Refugees	Student
Positive	"Thank you for providing information to a population that may have otherwise not received anything." "The partnership with the university helps us dream big and involve individuals that otherwise are not interested in refugees in our city." "The program provides services that we do not have resources for. At the same time students get to learn in a real-world setting. It's a win/win!" "Innovative; sustainable program!"	"My favorite part of the Fair is that my kids know more about health and healthy food." "I will tell my people to come and attend the next event." "The session helped me understand why I may need to have a flu-shot." "It's a really good experience for me to get to know more about health, improve my health." "I respect the students who care about me."	"It has really opened my eyes to refugees in Omaha to better understand the various challenges they face." "The most important part was to gain trust and build relationships with strangers: refugees and other health profession students." "I developed appreciation and awareness to the notion that nothing should be taken for granted." "I learned how important is cultural awareness and competent cultural practice."
Negative	"Shorten refugee evaluations they are hard to understand." "Make sure you use language that is simple and clear."	"They ran out of flu shots and I didn't get one!" "I want them to offer more dental care and glasses."	"I need more cultural training to be effective." "Needed interpreters, but lacked sufficient funding."

For example, following each health fair, refugees are asked to complete an oral evaluation. Of the 350 refugees who attended the past Fair, 131 completed the survey of which 99% indicated that the event was 'most useful' (rated 10 on a scale of 1-10 the usefulness of the health fair - 1 being least useful and 10 being most useful), and that the information was presented in a way that they could understand. Additional responses from the refugees include the desire to have more clinical services offered and an indication of the variety of 'favorite booths' such as, basic health screenings, nutrition, over-the-counter medication, free vaccinations, dental care and vision screenings with eye glasses.

Student perspectives

With each health education session, students take part in a pre/post assessment to determine knowledge, skills, comfort, and beliefs of the student's cultural competency. The aggregate analysis of the pre and post assessments, administered to a total of 29 students over three consecutive sessions in 2013 with the Bhutanese population concluded the following in regard to knowledge, skills and cross cultural competence: following the cultural awareness training, 80% of students reported an *increase in knowledge* of cultural challenges that face refugees in U.S. and an *increase in skills* with student's ability to communicate effectively with different cultures regardless of race, ethnicity, culture or language (increase from 2 to 4 on a Likert scale [1-least, 5-most].

Students have also consistently reflected positively on their experiences through BTC. For example, following a Somali health education session, a student stated, "It has really opened my eyes to the refugee population in Omaha and the various challenges they face." Another student reflected "….It was a rewarding experience and I felt like I was doing something that really mattered for the community. The Bridge to Care organization is a great way to interact with the diverse community that lives within Omaha. It was very beneficial to learn about a different culture as well as use skills we have learned from our time at UNMC towards those in need. I will be able to use what I learned on Sunday for the rest of my career. I would encourage anyone to help out with a Bridge to Care event[s] because not only are you helping others, you are also bettering yourself as a person as well as a professional."

Discussion

The work with refugees has been often challenging, complex, and at the same time very rewarding. In various listening sessions during the past 2 years, refugees in Omaha identified the following needs: housing, health, employment, education, transportation and public safety/community awareness. Bridge to Care focused on healthcare issues, while taking into consideration the host of challenges the community face. The major lessons learned are listed below:

1. Understanding of U.S. healthcare system - many members of the American society struggle to fully understand the ins and outs of the U.S. healthcare system, especially at a time of major changes in insurance coverage. Refugees have little foundational understanding of this complex system and often fall victims to misunderstandings and incur startling costs for minor services obtained outside of insurance coverage or in an inappropriate manner (for example - use of ER for simple upper respiratory infection). Refugees hold a unique understanding of health and sickness, embracing a holistic approach to treatment of diseases (American medicine is deeply embedded upon scientific data and physical exam, when other cultures look at the environment, cultural customs and traditions, and rely heavily on healers for cures). The BTC program has to be both efficient in assisting the understanding of the healthcare system while maintaining sensitivity to the traditional approach when presenting strategies for diagnosis and management of diseases.

2. Understanding preventive care - Students learned firsthand how individuals from diverse populations, cultural practices and beliefs have very different perceptions and understanding regarding health. A striking example was preventive health services, discussed at an education session as an important part of maintaining good health. Yet, 'preventive care', regarding cancer in the Bhutanese community, was found to be a new concept and a problematic one: "if you talk about or schedule screening for colon or cervical cancer you will bring it upon yourself". BTC has learned that more education and time is needed for preventive practices to be understood and embraced by refugees. This finding was an important one that we shared with the practice clinical community.

3. Refugee participation in sessions: Almost all refugees, regardless of geographic location, tend to avoid drawing attention to themselves. Asian refugees, especially, tend to be quite reserved. This means remaining silent rather than speaking up, not asking questions, not asking for clarification and essentially agreeing with whatever is said or done. Because time is limited in the education sessions, it is difficult to check for understanding, to assess how much of the presented material is comprehended, and how useful it was for the refugees. With consistent repetition of health topics presented at health education sessions, the hope is that the information will eventually be absorbed.

4. Sensitive topics: Another challenge has been the discussion of more sensitive topics such as women's health, torture and abuse, mental illness and subjects related to sex (i.e. sexually transmitted diseases). Generally speaking, these topics are discussed very little in the community or in the home and special measures must be taken in order to successfully address them. Due to matters of sensitivity and confidentiality, interpreters coming from the community are especially unsuitable when discussing these personal issues. The interpreters need to correctly communicate the health needs of their respective populations, and be of an appropriate age with adequate knowledge. Medically-certified interpreters are in very high demand, and as a result, are quite expensive and often unavailable. Finding competent medical interpreters was a challenge for BTC as it was for the practice community, and many of the sensitive topics could not be addressed. New initiatives designed to address mental health and other sensitive topics in group settings are currently being developed.

5. Logistics of the program - The general logistics for the BTC program have been a challenge and a great lesson to all involved. Scheduling planning meetings, session dates/times, session venues, refugee recruitment and selecting appropriate food have all required on-going open communication, flexibility, leadership and good problem solving skills. Refugees often work the first (7-4) and second (2-10) shifts 6-7 days a week, have limited access to transportation, and prefer gatherings in places of worship or at the housing complexes where most of the community members live. Since weekends tend to work best for the refugees, the students, community organization leaders and faculty extended their commitment to meet these needs, scheduling most activities on the weekends. Several sessions have been held following the conclusion of an existing ESL class or after faith-based activities to reach a larger number of refugees. In addition, students from the various health professions have to coordinate between the various professional curricula to ensure student participation (avoiding dates prior to major exams etc.). In addition, for each activity, interpreters need to be recruited. They are expected to disseminate information about the activity, recruit individuals to attend, and be present at the session. As stated earlier, interpreters are in high demand and need to be contacted long in advance.

Timely communication has also been an enduring challenge; perhaps the different perception of 'time', the lack of access to electronic communication, or the difference in norms and expectations for follow-up and response. In any case, the expectation of prompt reply to phone messages and emails is unrealistic and adds another layer to coordination.

6. Funding and sustainability - Each of the BTC's activities, especially the bi-annual health fairs, require resources (i.e. medical supplies, transportation, food, translated materials, and many other relevant items). Funding for BTC activities has been secured through an ongoing effort by the SLA, through applications to local and national grants and for in-kind contributions. Since its inception in 2010, over $20,000 cash funding were secured with over $100,000 in-kind services. Although tedious and very time consuming, through this process, BTC has formed numerous partnerships with local businesses and service providers.

New opportunities: The Refugee Health Collaborative

As a direct result of the BTC program, the Nebraska Refugee Health Collaborative (RHC) was formed, with the goal to improve health of the refugees who are a part of the fabric of the community. Twelve organizations joined together: UNMC, College of Public Health, (including the Service Learning Academy and Bridge to Care), Southern Sudan Community Association, Lutheran Family Services, Embrace the Nations, Omaha Together One Community, Institute of Public Life, Nebraska Department of Health and Human Services (Refugee Coordinator and Refugee Health Coordinator), Douglas County Health Department, Ready in Five, Alegent-Creighton Florence Clinic, One World Community Health Centers, Omaha Public Schools, and to date, over 250 refugee leaders and key community members have participated in the monthly meetings.

Much like BTC, the larger RHC embraced the following goals: to develop mutual understanding and trust among the group, to determine major perceived barriers to service (i.e. economic, cultural, language, financial, organizational, navigation of the health system, insurance), to identify culturally appropriate methods of engagement and to determine priorities and opportunities for action.

There are two sub-committees working under the RHC. The first is the Engagement Team, which looks at methods of engaging the refugee community in order to build capacity, improve existing and develop new services and empower the targeted populations to improve their own health. The second is the Data Team, which works a) to help clarify the number of refugees and their respective culture groups living in Omaha. Existing data sources were identified and will be linked to create a usable database that will support future activities including engagement and research; b) to develop scientific research grant applications and secuire major funding to ensure the sustainability of BTC and the RHC. In addition, the RHC is diligently working to develop a community health worker program with the refugee communities. The RHC encourages refugee involvement at all levels including refugee leaders from all groups who are represented in the city. This is not merely a project; the RHC is committed to long-term goals and implementation. With diverse team members from academia, local refugee organizations and refugee community leaders, the potential for successful outcomes is promising.

As we identify and embrace the different refugee groups in Omaha NE, we can better understand health-related needs, develop effective interventions, enhance cultural sensitivity and track outcomes. All are bound to benefit from this endeavor.

Limitations

The limitations of this project center on the assessment of its effectiveness. Currently, due to language barriers, limited resources, slow coordination among agencies, and limited data-sharing agreements, we are unable to better track how the program is making a difference in the community. With a $50,000 grant recently obtained for linkage of data and the development of a comprehensive data system for the city, we hope to better capture the impact on health and other related outcomes in the near future.

Conclusion

The definition of Health as referred by the World Health Organization (WHO) is especially important when considering the refugee populations (13). Started in 2010 from an initiative of a caring student (author CN) the inter-professional student-led/community-engaged Bridge to Care project expanded its activities into 2014. It created great ripples for further collaborative action and capacity building to improve the health of the refugee community. Students are rewarded with an exceptional real-life community based experience, while community needs are addressed, local capacity is established, and sustainability is built.

Acknowledgments

We are deeply grateful for the work of all of the Bridge to Care student leaders and student volunteers, the faculty volunteers who supervise and mentor the students, the refugee community leaders; and to the refugee service organizations leaders and staff who trust and nurture this partnership.

References

[1] UNHCR: The UN Refugee Agency. A pocket guide to refugees 2008. URL: http://www.unhcr.org/pages/49c3646c4b8.html

[2] US Office of Refugee Resettlement. Refugee arrival data 2000-2012. URL: http://www.acf.hhs.gov/programs/orr/resource/refugee-arrival-data

[3] US Department of State Refugee Resettlement in the United States 2013. URL: http://www.state.gov/j/prm/releases/factsheets/2013/203578.htm

[4] Department of Health and Human Services-Nebraska, 2012-2013 Minority Health Initiative Annual Report. URL: http://dhhs.ne.gov/Pages/srd_srdindex.aspx

[5] Lainof CA, Elsea SJ. From Sudan to Omaha: how one community is helping African refugees find a new home. Am J Nurs 2004;104:58-61.

[6] Tompkins M, Smith L, Jones K, Swundell S. HIV-education needs among Sudanese immigrants and refugees in the midwestern United States. AIDS Behav 2006;10:319-23.

[7] Benner MT, Townsend J, Kaloi W, Htwe K, Naranichakul N, Hunnangkul S, et al. Reproductive health and quality of life of young Burmese refugees in Thailand. Confl Health 2010;4:5.

[8] Campbell DS. Health hazards in the meatpacking industry. Occup Med 1999;14(2):351-72.

[9] World Health Organization. Overcoming migrants' barriers to health. URL: http://www.who.int/bulletin/volumes/86/8/08-020808/en/

[10] Morris MD, Popper ST, Rodwell TC, Brodine SK, Brouwer KC. Healthcare barriers of refugees post-resettlement. J Commun Health 2009;34:529-38.

[11] Carswell K, Blackburn P, Barker C. The relationship between trauma post-migration problems and the psychological well-being of refugees and asylum seekers. Int J Soc Psychiatry 2011;57:107-19.

[12] Herrel N, Olevitch L, Dubois DK, Terry P, Thorp D, Kind E, el al. Somali refugee women speak out about their needs for care during pregnancy and delivery. J Midwifery Womens Health 2004;49:345-9.
[13] World Health Organization. Preamble to the Constitution of the World Health Organization 1946. URL: http://www.who.int/about/definition/en/print.html
[14] Israel BA, Schulz AJ, Parker EA, Becker AB. Review of community-based research: assessing partnership approaches to improve public health. Annu Rev Public Health 1998;19:173-202.

In: Public Health
Editors: Rosemary M. Caron and Joav Merrick

ISBN: 978-1-63321-569-6

Chapter 13

Homeless adolescents and perceptions of health care

Ricky T Munoz, JD, MSW*[*1], Jeremy S Aragon, MSW[2] and Mark D Fox, MD, PhD, MPH[1]

[1]Center for Health Outcomes and Improvement Research,
University of Oklahoma School of Community Medicine, Section of Medicine/Pediatrics,
Department of Pediatrics, University of Oklahoma School of Community Medicine and
[2]Anne and Henry Zarrow School of Social Work, University of Oklahoma, Tulsa,
Oklahoma, US

Research has demonstrated that homeless adolescents have poorer health than their housed counterparts. We theorize that poor health outcomes are partially related to the perceptions homeless adolescents have of receiving care and the adverse effects of those perceptions on health seeking behaviors. Objective: To report on homeless adolescents perceptions regarding obtaining health care and to use the data to expand care for the homeless adolescent community whom we sampled. Participants: English-speaking adolescents aged 16-24 years who were receiving services from a homeless adolescent outreach agency located in the south central United States. Methods: Community-engaged qualitative research consisting of semi-structured interviews and focus groups. The narrative data from our focus groups and individual interviews were analyzed for content that was grouped into themes. Results: 30 adolescents participated, with 21 electing focus groups and 9 electing individual interviews. Themes include 1) homeless adolescents report feeling dehumanized when receiving health care; 2) the dehumanizing effect is related to the profit driven structure of the US Health Care System; 3) homeless adolescents react to dehumanizing care by avoiding care or turning to informal care networks; and 4.) active efforts are needed by health care providers to gain the trust of homeless adolescents. Conclusion: The perception among homeless adolescents that receiving health care is dehumanizing may be a contributing factor to poorer health outcomes for this population. We conclude with a discussion of how we translated results into practice with our community of interest consistent with the principals of community engaged research.

* Correspondence: Ricky T Munoz, JD, MSW, University of Oklahoma – Tulsa, 4502 East 41st Street, Tulsa, Oklahoma 74135, United States. E-mail: rmunoz@ou.edu.

Introduction

According to the most recent US federal data, nearly 1.7 million adolescents annually experience a "runaway/thrownaway" episode, resulting in homelessness or placing them "at risk" for homelessness (1). It is well established that homelessness is associated with poorer health, with homeless adolescents exhibiting disproportionately higher rates of illegal substance abuse, sexually transmitted infections, unwanted pregnancies, mental illness, and insufficient access to health care than housed adolescents (2-6). Many of such poor health outcomes are a logical consequence of the conditions of homelessness, such as poor nutrition and hygiene, crowding, violence, and the need for survival sex (3,5).

The social and environmental determinants of poor health for homeless adolescents are complex, with comprehensive solutions being a matter of public policy beyond what can be affected solely in clinical settings. Nevertheless, despite the seemingly intransigent barriers to good health for homeless adolescents, we believe there is room for health care providers to mediate the impact of these barriers by creating better models of health care delivery. Our goal with our current effort was to use community engaged research to develop a testable theory on the relationship between the perceptions of homeless adolescents of health care delivery and the impact of those perceptions on homeless adolescents' health seeking behavior. Our goal was to create transferable principals that can be used by other practitioners in the development improved models of health care delivery uniquely suited for homeless adolescents.

Our project

We employed a community-engaged research model to engage homeless adolescents in contributing to the development of a new program for health care delivery to meet their unique needs. Community-engaged research has been championed as a method to further reduce health inequalities, (7) through emphasizing the development of lasting relationships between researchers and the community of interest (8,9).

To that end, we spent time throughout the research process cultivating a lasting relationship with the staff and clients of a street outreach program of a local social services agency.

Our goal from our community engaged approach was not simply to collect data; while data collection was important, we also wanted to simultaneously demonstrate our commitment to addressing health issues of the local homeless adolescent population through the development of programs that arose directly from our research. Thus, our data were intended to serve not only academic purposes, but to provide an immediate benefit to the homeless adolescents we sampled.

Sampling

Study participants included clients (ages 16-24 years) receiving services from the homeless adolescent program of a social services agency in medium-sized city in the south-central

United States. All participants were identified by the partnering agency as either homeless or "at risk" for homelessness. Potential participants were informed of the nature of the study and invited to participate in either focus groups or individual interviews based on individual preference. Participants were provided a consent information sheet that explained the the purpose of the study was to gauge the perceptions of homeless adolescents regarding health care for their community. Participants were offered a $10 gift card for their time and modest refreshments. Consent was expressed through their participation in either a focus group that lasted 60-90 minutes or an individual interview that ranged from 30-60 minutes. The study protocol was approved by the Institutional Review Board of the University of Oklahoma Health Sciences Center.

Focus groups and individual interviews were semi-structured to promote conversational, two-way communication (10). Researchers followed question guidelines based on community- and health-related themes, but were free to follow conversation trajectories based on topics that participating adolescents deemed significant. As part of our philosophy of community engagement, the question guides were reviewed by agency staff prior to implementation and agency staff participated in focus groups and interviews when they desired. All focus groups and interviews were conducted in English.

Thirty adolescents, 19 males and 11 females, met our sampling criteria and completed the study. Of those 30, 21 elected to participate in focus groups and 9 choose individual interviews. The mean age of participants was 20.3 years of age the gender make-up consisting of 65% male and 35% female. Race distribution was 50% White, 28% African American, 11% Multi-racial, 5% American Indian /Alaskan Native, 3% Hispanic, and 3% other.

Analysis

All focus groups and individual interviews were audio-recorded, transcribed, and supplemented by notes taken by the research team. Once transcription was completed, NVIVO software was used to perform a content analysis to group the narrative data into themes. The final decision regarding the total number of interviews was made according to the principal of saturation, with sampling discontinued once we made the judgment that no new themes were emerging (11). Results were then used to develop a testable theoretical model for future research (11).

Findings

A major theme was homeless adolescents' perceive a lack of respect from health care providers that comes from being poor and homeless. For instance, when asked about how well health care providers understood the unique health care needs and challenges for homeless patients, one focus group collectively burst into laughter, with a female participant capturing the group sentiment:

> It doesn't seem like they want to (laughter subsiding) ... I mean they don't care . . . most of the time because we go to the ER, they just want us in and out. They don't care to find out about the situation.

The following quote also indicates a perception that receiving health care is dehumanizing:

> I would rather see a doctor that cares more than go to the ER and be treated like you're the stupidest person on the planet, or a fungus,...treated like you have no intelligence at all...I'm better than you because I went to medical school.

Consistently, participants indicated that health care providers devalue their health care needs because they are homeless and poor.

Dehumanization is a systematic: "It's all about the money"

Participants were relatively aware of the structural challenges within the health care system associated with financing. A second major theme was profit-driven models of care leave no room for the needs of homeless adolescents. The following excerpts are exemplary of homeless adolescents who felt health care is "all about money":

> I was sitting there arguing with him over that it's not a sprain, it's broke and it's swelled up over twice its normal size...And because I didn't have insurance he was just telling me it was just sprained. He's going to wrap it with an ace wrap.
>
> They're gonna get the ones that's got insurance first and then you know they'll worry about the ones that don't, and I don't think it's right...

> I've actually had an ER doctor tell me 'You need this test but since you don't have insurance, we can do without it'...Their decisions are all based on money.

One participant was even aware of the concept of "single payer" model, and suggested a health care financing model like the one in "France" is needed to help reduce health disparities.

The impact of perceptions on health seeing behavior: "Toughing it out"

The perceptions that health care providers in the US dehumanize homeless adolescent because of the financial drivers of health delivery appears to influence homeless adolescent's health seeking behaviors. The following themes capture what homeless adolescent describe as their strategies for dealing with the perceived barriers to receiving good care noted above.

First, the desire to avoid unpleasant interactions with health care providers contributes to homeless adolescents' reluctance to seek care, which one described as the "toughing it out" approach to better health. A female homeless adolescent's comment epitomizes this view:

> If we can't pay, we can't afford it, so we don't go unless it's a major emergency. Unless there is really something wrong ... If you're puking up blood then yeah, you need to go to the hospital. I've got bad ankles... If those are hurting, oh well, they've been hurting for two weeks. If I can't stand them anymore then I need to go to the hospital. So it's deal with it until you have no other choice.

Further, to reduce the need to seek care from an insensitive, formal health care delivery system, homeless adolescents in our sample reported turning to informal peer networks for alternative care. For example, one male participant shared:

> Well, me, I'm probably different than most people … I can take and make splints; I know how to splint my fingers. I can splint my arm if I really had to, if it's broken. Basically I do the best I can, if somebody I know needs help, or if they've broke their leg or ankle, I help them.

Respondents who reported turning to other homeless adolescents for health care also reported a sense of community that increases their trust for those in their informal peer networks.

Solutions from a homeless adolescent perspective: "Be a little more understanding"

Although homeless adolescents exhibited distrust of health of the health care system, participants also held hope that health care delivery could be improved. For instance, one female homeless adolescent suggested more egalitarian partnerships with providers that incorporate shared decision making would help increase trust:

> Be a little more understanding…At least consider some of my ideas in the treatment plan instead of shoving me off like I don't know what I'm talking about. I don't know everything just like he don't know everything, you know, but the difference is I can admit it.

Another homeless male adolescent described a particular encounter he had with a health care provider during which the provider valued his perspective and incorporated it into the care plan:

> I went to the hospital because I couldn't deal with the pain anymore, and the first time in my entire life, I had a doctor actually look at me and go, what kind of medicine do you want?…that's the first time I ever had them ask my opinion. There's a doctor that cares…

While deliberate efforts to better engage homeless adolescent will not change the financing model of the US health care system, such practice improvements may have a degree of positive impact on homeless adolescents' perceptions and their associated health seeking behaviors.

Community engaged research as relationship building

A key element of community engaged research is to use data collection as a means to build lasting relationship with study participants (9). In our case, data collection allowed for the strengthening of a social connection between the researchers and the homeless adolescent being studied. We found evidence of this with reports from homeless adolescents that they appreciated the opportunity to have their opinions heard, with one adolescent stating "You seem different, like you care about what we think". This response was brought on by the engagement associated with the research effort, which opened a door to us to further a clinical relationship with the homeless adolescents. The positive response to our data collection efforts suggests that homeless adolescents' negative perceptions of health care providers are not dispositional traits; rather, such perceptions are subject to interventions that build trust and encouragingly, community engaged research can be such an intervention.

Discussion

Our results add to the literature by producing results similar to other research that shows that the interpersonal aspect of health care delivery is important to homeless adolescents (12-13). More specifically, our study makes generalizability claims stronger on conclusions that homeless adolescents feel dehumanized by the health care system (12-13). Our research also adds to the literature by offering a theoretical link between perceptions of dehumanizing care and health care seeking behaviors of homeless adolescents.

Theory development

While a portion of our current study reinforces earlier findings, the strength of qualitative research is that it offers the opportunity to create testable hypotheses. In our case, our data suggests a theoretical model for poorer health outcomes for homeless adolescents that traces to perceptions by homeless adolescents of health care providers. Our model begins with the perceptions of homeless adolescents that health care providers do not respect them for financial reasons. Because of this perception, the resulting behaviors of homeless adolescents include avoidance of health care and/or the utilization of informal peer networks of care. We hypothesize the end result of the relationship between these variables is poorer health as depicted in Figure 1.

Before continuing, in the United States it is important to note that Patient Protection and Affordable Care Act (PPACA) expands insurance opportunities for homeless adolescents in some states (14).

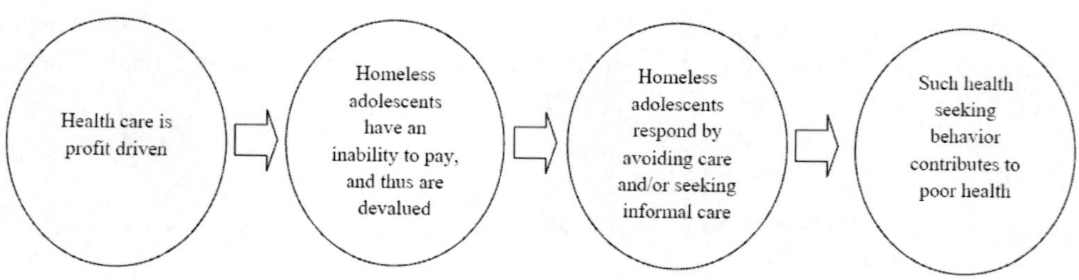

Figure 1. Proposed Relationship Model of Poorer Health Outcomes for Homeless Adolescents Based on their Perceptions of Health Care Delivery (N = 30).

In the state in which the research was conducted, that had not yet occurred at the time of writing. However, this disparity in expanded access does offer an opportunity for comparison research to determine if homeless adolescents' in states that have expanded insurance opportunities exhibit changes in perceptions of the health care system associated with the possession of health insurance. It may be that the introduction of health insurance moderates the relationship between the variables we depict in our model.

Ongoing community engagement

An additional contribution to the literature by our study is a description of how community engaged research can be used to build a lasting relationship with a community of interest. We think effective community engaged research involves approaching the research with a commitment to the principal of *reciprocity*, meaning a commitment by the researchers to return to the community a tangible benefit in exchange for their time (15). To do otherwise could be considered a form of *academic imperialism*, reminiscent of archaeologists of old that carried artifacts from exotic places back to their homelands for display without tangible return to the community from which the artifacts were obtained (15). To offer guidance on how we delivered reciprocity in our study, we elected to also report how our research effort directly contributed to ongoing relationships between the research team, the agency, and the homeless adolescents we seek to serve better.

Expansion of clinical activities

At the local level of our community of interest, the data was used to obtain grant funding to expand clinic services to the homeless adolescents population from which our sample was drawn. In this way, the data was used to further a lasting relationship with the community. Moreover, the practices outlined in the following paragraphs describe how results were used to inform our clinic's practice models for better service to the local homeless adolescent community.

As noted above, several participants reported that the act of interacting through interviews was a trust-building exercise. Carrying this model into our clinical practice, we now deliberately spend time conversing with homeless adolescents in locations they frequent, such as the homeless adolescent "drop-in" area located near our clinic. The goal is to interact with homeless adolescents in an egalitarian, non-clinical manner in comfortable social environments that promotes increased trust (16). Furthermore, the egalitarian communication style that starts outside the clinic continues once adolescents enter. We minimize the interactions that occur "across the exam table," through learning the adolescents' preferred street names and engaging in social conversations (16). Our clinic staff also dresses informally to create a relaxed, collegial environment designed to reduce the psychological barrier between provider and homeless adolescents (16).

An additional element of research team incorporated into the clinic includes the use of community health workers (CHWs) (17). CHWs are members of the clinic staff that are drawn from the homeless adolescent population. We based our CHW program on respondents' reports that they feel comfortable turning to peers for assistance. As of this writing, we have two members of the community who work with us to help homeless adolescents navigate the clinic and the health care system more broadly.

Limitations and future research

The limitations of our study are those found in all qualitative research, in that our small sample does not allow for a statistical generalization of our results to the entire population of homeless adolescents. Despite that limitation, our study adds to a developing body of research on homeless adolescents' and health care by offering a testable theory of the linkage between homeless adolescents' perceptions of health care providers, health seeking behavior, and health outcomes. While it is certain that ecological variables such as a lack of adequate nutrition, housing, stress, etc. play a significant role in producing poor health care outcomes for homeless adolescents, future research should explore how much of a contribution poor perceptions of health care providers makes to health seeking behaviors for homeless adolescents and how those health seeking behaviors affect health outcomes. Our research also suggests a need for additional intervention research to test specific practice models to determine exactly which qualify as best practices for reducing distrust by homeless adolescents of the health care delivery system.

Conclusion

Our community engaged research approach collected qualitative data that suggests homeless adolescents' health access behaviors are driven by their negative perceptions of their treatment by health care providers and that these health seeking behaviors may be a contributor to poorer health outcomes for this population. Our approach also met the twin aims of community engaged research of not only producing data that is transferable to other health care providers, but also reciprocating to the community being studied by expanded clinical services based on the data and relationships made via the research. We are honored to have the opportunity to work with the homeless adolescent participants in our study and believe that similar research models in other communities will help realize the goals of reducing health disparities like those experienced by the homeless adolescents of our community.

Acknowledgments

Our research was supported by the National Center for Research Resources and the National Institute of General Medical Sciences of the National Institutes of Health through Grant Number 8P20GM103447. The authors also would like to acknowledge Cordell Baker, BS, for his assistance with this research. All authors certify that we have no conflicts of interest in relation to this study.

References

[1] Hammer H., Finkelhor D, Sedlak AJ. National incidence studies of missing, abducted, runaway, and thrownaway children. Runaway/thrownaway children: National estimates and characteristics. [Internet]. Washington, DC, US: Department of Justice, Office of Justice Programs, Office of Juvenile Justice and Delinquency Prevention, 2002. URL: https://www.ncjrs.gov/pdffiles1/ojjdp/196469.pdf.

[2] Ammerman SD, Ensign J, Kirzner R, Meininger ET, Tornabene M, Warf CW, Zerger S, Post P. Homeless young adults 18-24: Examining service delivery adaptations. [Internet]. Nashville, TN, US: National Health Care for the Homeless Council, 2004. URL: http://www.nhchc.org/Publications/younghomelessadult1.pdf.

[3] Feldmann J, Middleman AB. Homeless adolescents: common clinical concerns. Semin Pediatr Infect Dis 2003;14:6–11.

[4] Nyamathi AM, Christian, A, Windokun F, Jones T, Strehlow A, Shoptaw S. Hepatitis C virus infection, substance use and mental illness among homeless youth: a review. AIDS 2005;19(Suppl 3):S34–S40.

[5] Rew L, Taylor-Seehafer M, Fitzgerald ML. Sexual abuse, alcohol, and other drug use, and suicidal behaviors in homeless adolescents. Issues Compr Pediatr Nurs 2001;24:225–40.

[6] Roy E, Haley N, Leclerc P, et al. Mortality in a cohort of street youth in Montreal, JAMA 2004;292:569-74.

[7] Schmittidiel J, Grumbach K, Selby J. System based participatory research in health care: an approach for sustainable research and quality. Ann Fam Med 2010;8(3):256-9.

[8] Lasker RD, Weiss ES. Broadening participation in community problem solving: a multidisciplinary model to support collaborative practice and research. J Urban Health 2003;80(1):14-47.

[9] Mulligana M, Nadarajah, Y. Working on the sustainability of local communities with a "community-engaged" research methodology. Local Environ Int J Justice Sustain 2008;13(2):81-94.

[10] Lindlof, TR, Taylor, BC. Qualitative communication research methods, 2nd ed. Thousand Oaks, CA: Sage, 2002.

[11] Patton MQ. Qualitative research and evaluation methods. Thousand Oaks, CA: Sage, 2002.

[12] Ensign, J. Quality of health care: the views of homeless youth. Health Serv Res 2004;39: 695–708.

[13] Hudson AL, Nyamathi A, Greengold B, Slagle A, Koniak-Griffin D, Khalilifard F, Getzoff D. Health-seeking challenges among homeless youth. Nurs Res 2010;59:212-8.

[14] Rudowitz, R. & Stephens, J. Analyzing the Impact of State Medicaid Expansion Decisions. [Internet]. Washington, DC: The Henry J. Kasier Family Foundation, 2013. URL: http://kff.org/medicaid/issue-brief/analyzing-the-impact-of-state-medicaid-expansion-decisions/.

[15] Glazer, M. The threat of the stranger: Vulnerability, reciprocity, and fieldwork. In: Sieber, J, ed. Ethics of social research: fieldwork, regulation, and publication. New York: Springer, 1982:49-70.

[16] Barry PJ, Ensign J, Lippek SH. Embracing street culture: fitting health care into the lives of street youth. J Transcult Nurs 2002;13:145-52.

[17] Martin M, Hernandez O, Naureckas E, Lantos J. Improving asthma research in an inner-city Latino neighborhood with community health workers. J Asthma 2005;42(10):891-9.

In: Public Health
Editors: Rosemary M. Caron and Joav Merrick
ISBN: 978-1-63321-569-6

Chapter 14

Community-centered design as a catalyst for change

Peter J Ellery*, BEd, MA, MLA, PhD[1], Jane Ellery, BS, MA, PhD[1], John Motloch, BArch, MLA, PhD[2] and Martha Hunt, BA, BLA, MLA[2]
[1]Fisher Institute for Wellness & Gerontology
[2]Department of Landscape Architecture, Ball State University, Muncie, Indiana, US

Universal Primary Education (UPE) in Uganda has resulted in a significant increase in student enrollment and the need for more teaching resources and infrastructure, especially in rural areas of the country. While more classrooms and schools are being built to address these needs, little attention has been directed toward the value of the landscape that surrounds school buildings. The purpose of this project was to use a community-centered, collaborative design approach to explore the potential of the landscape surrounding a school. Site concept plans and images were developed in collaboration with school participant groups consisting of students, teachers, the School Management Committee, and local community members for the Building Tomorrow (BT) Lutiisi Academy primary school in Wakiso, Uganda. These plans and images highlighted potential health and educational opportunities that exist within the landscape surrounding this school and allowed school participant groups to envision the school as being more than just a building or classrooms. The plans and images were further explored, discussed, and revised by the school participant groups. These combined efforts resulted in the community committing the financial and human resources needed for the construction of new teacher housing on the site.

* Correspondence: Peter J. Ellery, BEd, MA, MLA, PhD, Fisher Institute for Wellness and Gerontology, Health and Physical Activity Building – HP 302/Room 305, Ball State University, Muncie, IN 47306, United States. E-mail: pellery@bsu.edu.

Introduction

One of the primary focal points in the United Nations Millennium Development Goals (UNMDG) is the reduction in the number of children in Africa who are uneducated by the year 2015 (1,2). In support of this goal, the Ugandan Government introduced legislation in 1997 that mandated Universal Primary Education (UPE) (1,3). This legislation ensures the right of every child in Uganda to a free Primary School level education and is based on the premise that education provides the nation with the literacy skills, income, health, political participation, liberty, and general welfare attributes essential to the political, social, and economic growth of Uganda as a nation (4).

In the year following the implementation of UPE, enrollment in government-owned primary schools increased by 58%. Enrollment figures at the primary school level have now stabilized and average? 86% of all children who are eligible to attend primary school (5). This rapid increase in government primary school enrollment, however, has created a significant strain on existing schools, teachers, teaching resources, drinking water, and hygienic latrine facilities. These resources are essential if children are to successfully complete their primary education and a significant concern for schools in rural areas of the country where funding for new construction or school improvements is less prevalent. More schools and schooling infrastructure are needed if the health and educational issues now being faced by the nation's primary school system are to be resolved (3,6).

In response to these concerns, externally funded organizations and foundations, like Building Tomorrow (BT) in the United States, have begun supporting the development and construction of more school buildings and infrastructure in rural areas of Uganda. Since its inception in 2006, BT has successfully built and opened 15 new primary schools, with a further five primary schools either in the site planning or construction phases of development. Each of these schools provides teaching and learning space for 325 primary school aged students, and BT has made a public commitment to the construction of 60 more primary schools by 2016. Key to the success of BT is the development of these primary schools in partnership with the community in which the school will be located. While BT is responsible for raising the money that will pay for the construction of the school, the community is responsible for the provision of the land, the construction of the school itself, and the maintenance and continued upkeep of the school once it has been completed. As BT notes, when a community partnership approach is used, "each school serves as a source of pride and a catalyst for change within the community. We have seen roads built, gardens harvested, scholarships funded, teachers organized, and housing constructed as a direct result of communities being empowered to help themselves (7)."

While organizations like BT are working effectively to build more school facilities and buildings in rural areas of Uganda, few have utilized the potential educational, health, and social opportunities the landscape surrounding the school can provide. This consideration of the landscape is perhaps even more important as many of the educational goals sought in the Ugandan primary school curriculum are ideally suited to a practical, outdoor learning environment (8–10). Further, research has shown that education in outdoor and natural settings can have a number of benefits including increased environmental knowledge, increased environmentally appropriate behavior, improved academic performance, and gains in physical health (11–15).

From a design thinking perspective, the landscape can be used to resolve health and educational issues that currently exist, while adding elements that support and supplement the school's mission and purpose (16,17). The additional land at a school, if designed effectively, could be used to harvest water, grow food, keep animals, house teachers, collect energy, and provide recreational space for both the children attending the school and the community surrounding it. The landscape could also promote learning opportunities through the creation of outdoor learning environments (18), and improve the appeal of the school for students, community members, and teachers through the addition of play and recreational facilities. With a significant portion of the primary school curriculum now focused on education in agriculture, community service, and health and physical education (10), the design of the school's landscape should be as important as the design and construction of the school building itself. In response to these issues, this study explored the potential of the school landscape to determine if it could be designed to better serve the needs of the students, teachers, and community members in that area.

The lutiisi academy primary school project

The site chosen for this project was the Lutiisi Academy primary school in Wakiso, Uganda. The school is located approximately 25 miles, or 40 kilometres, north west of Kampala along the Kampala-Hoima road. The Lutiisi Academy was the first school to be built by BT. It was selected for this project because it could be accessed from Kampala on a daily basis, it was approximately 6.5 acres in size, and it had been completed and in operation since 2006. This last factor was particularly important because it meant the school had students, teachers, and a well-established, community-based School Management Committee that could also take part in this design initiative.

The study utilized a participatory approach (19) that was designed to engage the BT staff, and school participant groups like students, teachers, the Lutiisi Academy School Management Committee, and local community members in discussions about the school's landscape (20,21). Information collected through personal discussions with the BT staff indicated they focused on school building construction and had yet to consider the role the land around the school. As such, they had no specific goals or issues that needed to be addressed but were interested to see what options might be available to them in the design and construction of future schools. Interviews were conducted with the principal and individual teachers at the school, and a focus group discussion was conducted with the School Management Committee and local community members. Notes and comments from teachers during the interview process were recorded directly as all of the teachers were able to communicate very well in English. Notes and comments from the School Management Committee and community member focus group discussion were recorded with the assistance of a translator. A translator was needed as the community members in attendance primarily spoke the local tribal language of the district, and not English. Data gathered from interviews and the group discussion were then analyzed to determine themes that could be addressed through design.

Students used an art-based activity to provide information regarding their play and recreational preferences for the school (22). This activity started with students from the school's year five (i.e., P5) class viewing images depicting a wide variety of play and recreational settings. They were then given the opportunity to discuss and draw what they would like to see as play and recreational areas at their school. Upon completion of their artwork, the students were videoed holding their pictures and describing in English what they had drawn. The student narratives were transcribed, and a word analysis showcased which terms were used most often to describe their play settings (23). The most commonly occurring terms were also identified as themes to be addressed in the design process.

The themes obtained from the teacher interviews and the School Management Committee and community member focus group discussion were combined with those from the children's art activity to develop a design program containing prioritized goals and objectives for the design process. A series of design iterations were developed to examine design opportunities for the school site. From these iterations, a concept site plan for the school was developed. This initial plan was shared with students, teachers, the School Management Committee, and community members from the school. These participants were encouraged to see the site concept plan as a starting point for discussion and revision of the design elements being suggested and to consider the feasibility of these elements actually being developed and implemented at the Lutiisi Academy primary school.

Data collection and analysis from interviews with school teachers

Teachers at the Lutiisi Academy Primary School were interviewed to determine their perspectives on how the school and school landscape could be improved. The teacher interview guide consisted of 25 open-ended questions. These questions covered topics like: (1) the role of education in preparation of children for life in Uganda; (2) the school as a work environment; (3) the school teaching day as it is experienced by teachers; (4) the physical working conditions at the school; (5) the problems teachers encounter in the school; (6) those aspects of the school they felt needed improvement; (7) what they would like to see added to the school; and (8) whether they would use the school facilities if there were adult educational or in-service programs made available to them through the school.

Information was obtained from four teachers through personal interviews during lunch and non-instructional times of the day. Examples of teacher comments included:

> "We don't have a lot of equipment or play things like swings or climbing apparatus. The children do have some sporting equipment to play formal games and they play these games in the small, grassed areas alongside the school. When they play sports formally, they have to go to another place that has a full size soccer field or sport space."
>
> "Everything from basic planting of plants, watering, making a garden, compost, mulching, herbicides and spraying for disease, etc. fertilizer are taught at the school. We don't have any livestock education involving animals like goats, pigs, or chickens, because you would need someone to watch for them during the holidays or at times when school is not in session."
>
> "We collect rainwater in a tank for drinking and compost vegetation and scraps for recycling and use on crops. We treat our water by boiling it on sheets of shiny corrugated iron for 12 hours in plastic bottles. This is needed because the water tank (2000 L) tank can only provide water for a week or two before being empty. When the water tank is dry, the water we drink comes from a well. It is not a deep well and the water is not very tasty or clean. It undergoes the same process of boiling to make it fit to drink."

"The latrines are 'dry' latrines (i.e., holes in the ground that will require the moving of the latrine in time). We are lucky though in that holidays and times when the children are not at school, the waste recedes extending the life of the latrine location. We would like to have a septic tank system as there is a government service that will come and empty it. We would also like a larger set of restrooms for both boys and girls and for them to be separate rather than joined by a common wall."

An analysis of the responses taken from the teachers who were interviewed produced the following themes:

1) The children need playgrounds, sporting fields and equipment.
2) Teachers need to be housed on school grounds.
3) Barriers are needed to keep neighboring livestock off school property.
4) Agricultural experiences involving animals, the environment, and energy issues need to be developed.
5) More water collection, storage and cleaning features are needed to increase water availability during dry periods.
6) Pit latrines need to be replaced with a septic tank toilet system, with separate facilities for teachers, male, and female students.
7) Power to the school is needed for lighting and the use of educational technologies.

Data collection and analysis from focus group discussions with the school management committee and community area parents

The School Management Committee along with interested community members were invited to be part of a focus group discussion to determine issues and concerns they would like to see addressed at the school. The discussion guide for the school management committee and community members consisted of 11 open ended questions. The topics addressed in this group discussion included: (1) the role of the school within the community; (2) a description of a regular day for the children attending the school; (3) a description of the educational areas being taught to their children; (4) their overall opinion of the school's instruction, the teachers and the school as it relates to their children's education; (5) the kinds of things they would like to see added or changed at the school; and, (6) whether they would use the school facilities if adult educational or recreational programs were available to them at the school.

Information was obtained from 15 participants, some of whom had walked three miles to attend the meeting. Responses were translated into English by local BT staff and examples of the comments made by participants during the meeting included:

"We want our children to pass these basic educational skills so that they can have a skill for the future like being a teacher, or a radio presenter, etc."

"If I die and left my child 10 acres of land, and they could not farm it, then they would just sell it and take the money. This money would just last a short time. But, if they had farming knowledge, they could then farm the land and grow things. The land now has personal as well as family value to the new family owner and now has on-going value and worth to them."

"I would like my children to learn about the agriculture of their community and the heritage-based, traditional methods that the community uses" (i.e., agricultural strategies that include permaculture techniques, mulching and composting, crop rotation, and other sustainable land management practices.)

"We would like to see the school have spaces for sports like Netball, Soccer, Track and Field Athletics, Boxing, Volleyball, Basketball, and Swimming", and "more playgrounds and play equipment like swings, climbing apparatus, and slides for the children."

An analysis of the School Management Committee and Community Member responses from the participants who took part in the focus group discussion produced the following themes:

1) The school curriculum needs to be extended to include livestock, issues related to permaculture, and sustainable farming practices.
2) More water collection is needed for drinking, sanitation, and instruction in health-related behaviors and practices.
3) Playgrounds are needed for child development, and sporting fields are needed for classes like physical education and school sporting teams.
4) More plants need to be grown for food and aesthetic appeal.
5) Teachers should be housed on the school grounds, and the school should be painted school colors.
6) The school needs electricity or a power source for lighting or teaching equipment.
7) The community should be able to use the school facilities.

Data collection and analysis obtained from the student artwork and video narration activity

Students from the Lutiisi Academy's P5 classes (i.e, students approximately 10 and 11 years of age) drew pictures of the play spaces they wanted at their school. Each then described their picture while being recorded on video. Each child's video narration was then transcribed. A word count and Wordle graphic were used to identify commonly occurring terms and themes expressed by the students (see Figure 1). Examples of student artwork descriptions include:

"I have drawn a flower, I like to teaching poetry, and to playing netball, swimming pool, and swing." The student is asked, "What is the animal the children are sitting on in the picture?" The student responds, "a crocodile."

"I have drawn the shed, I have drawn the swing, I have drawn (the word cannot be understood from the recording but the child is pointing to the climbing wall)." The student is asked, "Why do you want a shelter?" The student responds, "eating porridge."

"I have drawn pictures of playing football, I have drawn a swings, I have drawn a people who are here (the student gestures to the children walking on a log)."

"I draw a swing, a flower, and a shed for drinking porridge to have for lunch."

"I have drawn a swing and fruit, a girl playing and a Uganda flag."

"The picture is of playing football. This is the goal keeper, this is the swing, this is the flag. The swing as at the top and at the bottom is a bulb – electricity, it is a light bulb."

"My name is Musisi and I want flowers for our compound. I want to see them. I want the flowers to be a border for the compound."

Analysis of the pictures, Wordle, and responses obtained from all of the children resulted in a number of playground elements being identified as needed for the school. These included:

1) The provision of a sporting field for games, physical education and sports like soccer, netball, volleyball.
2) The creation of play spaces with recreation equipment that includes swings, slides and climbing apparatus.
3) The addition of trees and flowers so the school is more aesthetically pleasing.
4) The addition of a shelter for shade and protection from the rain with seating and tables for lunch and getting together to talk as a group.

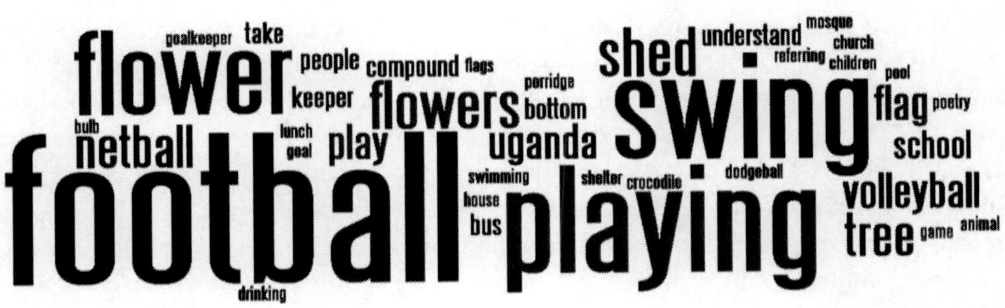

Figure 1. "Wordle", or graphical depiction of the 30 most used words used in the narratives given by students when describing their drawings (*Note: The more a word is repeated in the transcript, the larger it appears in the Wordle.

Physical site analysis of the Lutiisi Academy property

The school property site was evaluated for physical terrain, vegetation, water runoff patterns, transportation routes, current use, and topography. This analysis included an evaluation of current and potential issues with the site's current configuration and the identification of potential spaces that would be well suited to the suggestions made by students, teachers, and community members. The property was also evaluated at a regional and national level for soil type and quality, climate, and population. These evaluations indicated that the school was located on primarily Ferralitic and acidic (i.e., low Ph value) soil. This type of soil is dense making drainage, surface runoff, and topsoil erosion a problem in clear cut areas on slopes, but it is excellent for agriculture and for the production of food crops like plantains, coffee, tea, citrus fruit, cocoa and rubber.

Uganda lies on the equator making the climate ideal for agriculture. The average daylight time is just over 12 hours per day, varying only 15 to 30 minutes over the year, and the region experiences an average of 6 hours of direct sunlight each day making it ideal for solar energy initiatives. In contrast, however, the climate found in Wakiso includes a bimodal rain season that increases the potential for drought if rainfall is below average and an increased likelihood of crop failure.

Uganda's population distribution is most dense around major cities and along transportation corridors. While the population density in the city of Kampala is greater than 500 people per square mile, the population density in the rural central plain area is only around 50 to 75 people per square mile. The Lutiisi Academy lies on the edge of the plain area where the population is low and spread over a wide area. It should be noted that some students live two to three miles away from the Lutiisi Academy, and it is not uncommon for children living in rural areas of Uganda to spend up to 90 minutes walking to and from school each day as there is little funding or support for school student transportation.

Findings

The themes established from the data analysis were used to develop a design program (i.e., a list of goals and objectives that are met through the design process) (see Table 1). A series of conceptual design iterations were generated to study options that could address these goals and objectives through effective landscape design. These iterations were evaluated and consolidated into a final site concept plan for the school (see Figure 2 and 3). Design elements that address the themes and concerns identified by the students, teachers, and community members are identified on the site concept plan and have been explained further in Table 2. A series of site sections and perspective renderings were also developed to accompany the site concept plan to show how these proposed changes to the landscape might appear when completed.

Table 1. Design program for the Lutiisi Academy Primary School

Goal 1: • Provide recreational spaces and amenities around the school that serve students, teachers and community member needs. **Design Objectives:** • Develop a sporting field area approximately 300 feet by 170 feet as a multisport playing field in close proximity to the school. • Identify and develop play areas for children of different age groups. • Provide a covered space that can be used for recreational and lunch purposes. • Provide new toilets and change rooms to support the recreational areas. • Provide additional flowerbeds, trees and vegetation to improve the aesthetic around the play areas.
Goal 2: • Increase the collection and amount of water available to the school. **Design Objectives:** • Include water tanks and roof rainwater collection with every building on the site.

• Increase the number of water tanks used at the school to ensure the school is independent of well water needs. • Include a solar hot water treatment process for water that is used for drinking and cooking purposes. • Include a solar powered pump system for the solar hot water system.
Goal 3: • Add trees and vegetation to slow water runoff from the site and increase aquifer recharge. **Design Objectives:** • Utilize permaculture and farming techniques that detain and hold water to slow runoff from the site. • Utilize hedged shrubs for living borders and fencing • Include an orchard and more fruit bearing trees in the landscape to increase food production on the school site as well as re-vegetate the site.
Goal 4: • Provide an appropriate septic human waste disposal system for teachers and students at the school. **Design Objectives:** • Design and locate toilets that are located near key teacher, student, and community use areas, and that can meet the needs of community, teachers and students. • Design and locate a septic well system for the toilets that can be easily accessed and emptied by government sanitation trucks if necessary.
Goal 5: • Expand and develop the agricultural potential of the landscape. **Design Objectives:** • Provide design options that address concerns related to soil erosion and flooding around the school building itself. • Provide livestock options for both instruction and food production services. • Provide on-site teacher housing that allows for teachers to be present and monitor the animals and crops during times when school is not in session. • Define on-site teacher crop spaces for teacher gardens and livestock accommodation.

Goal 6:
• Provide a renewable energy source and energy storage system for the school.
Design Objectives:
• Provide enough roofing Solar Panels to the school roof and surrounding buildings to create electrical energy for:
  o for the lighting of a single classroom; and,
  o the power needs of 10 computer systems for approximately 4 hours.
• Ensure solar panels are included as part of all new buildings (i.e., latrines, kitchen, etc.) for lighting, pumping water, etc.

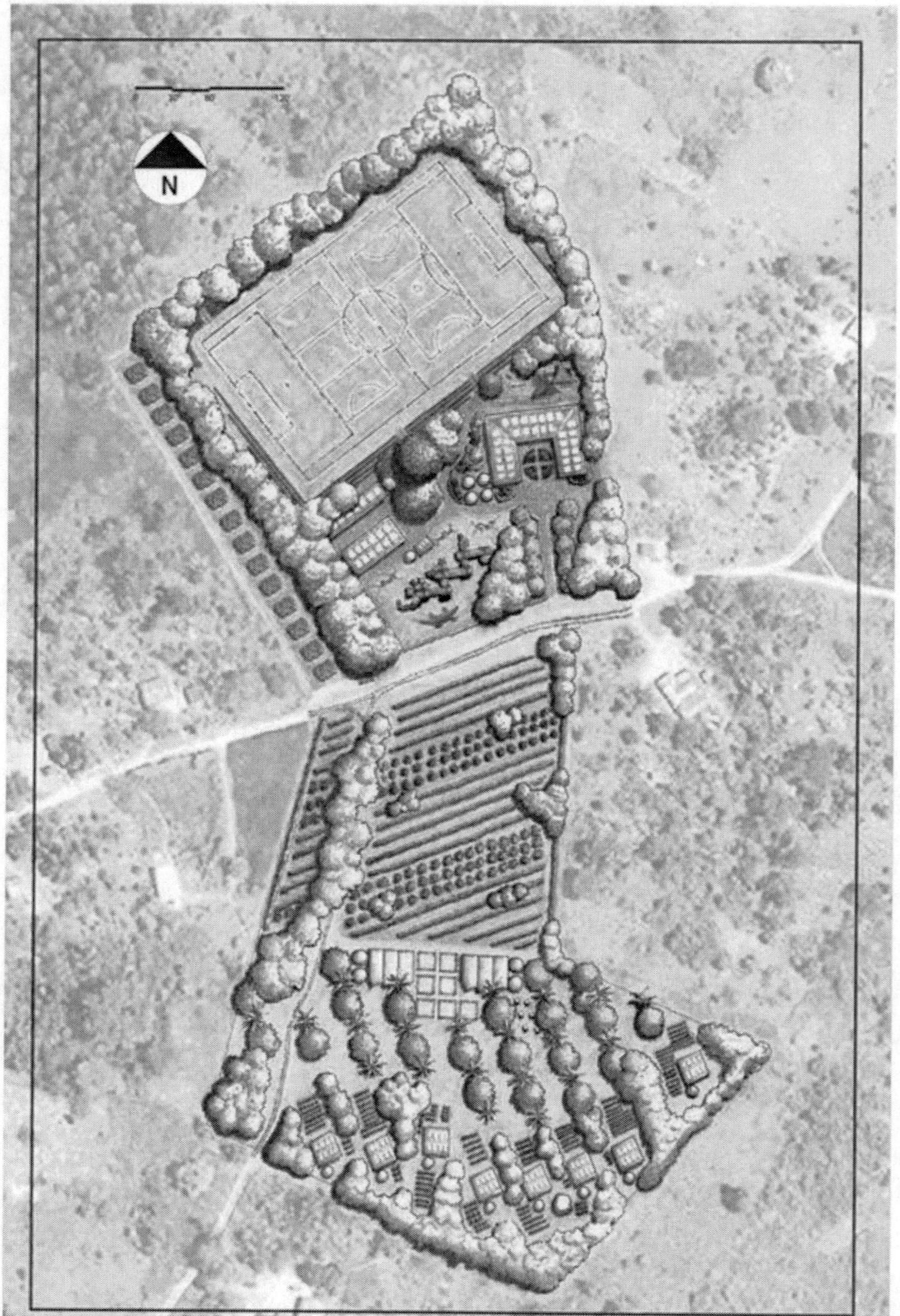

Figure 2. Aerial photo overlay of Lutiisi Academy Primary School site concept plan.

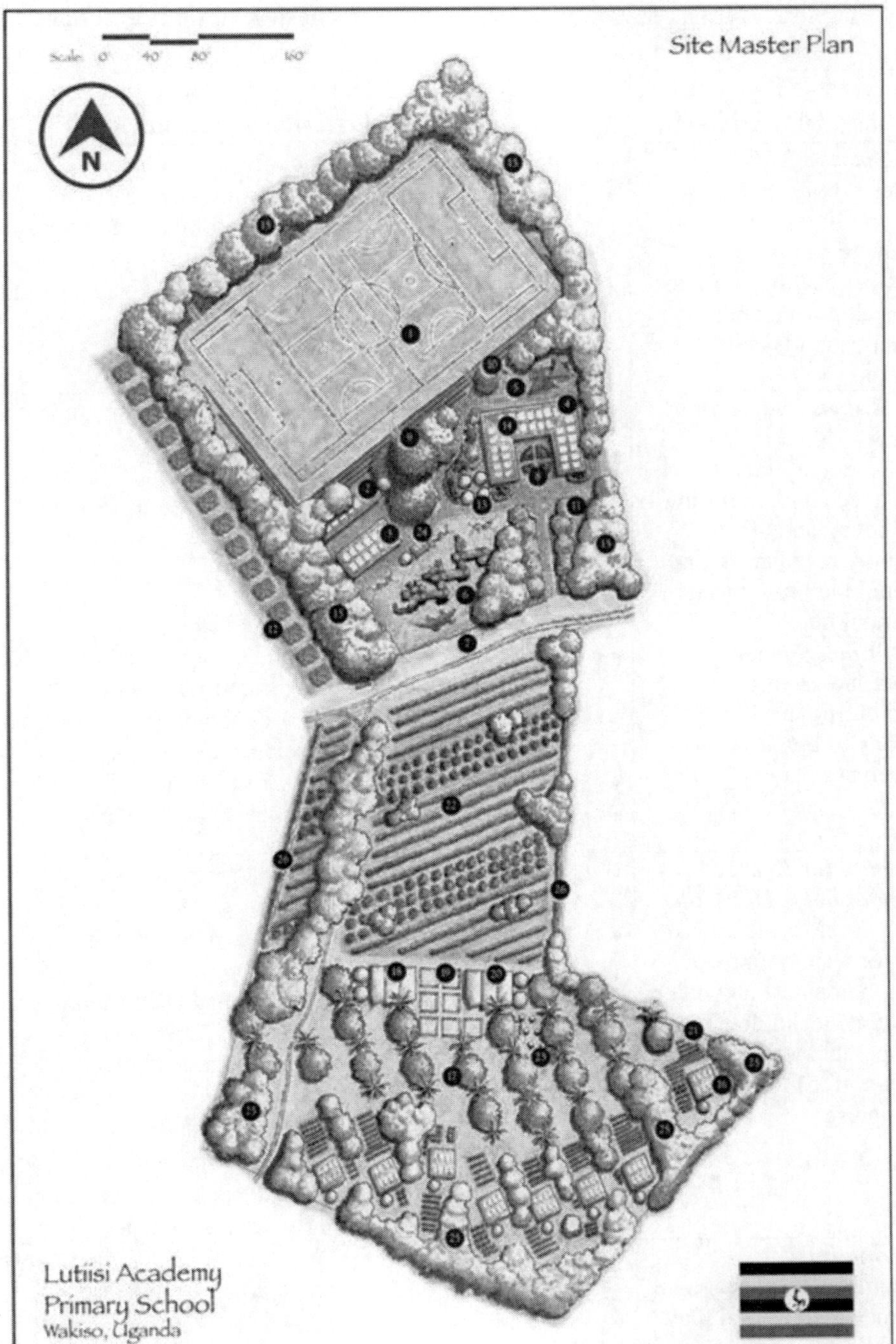

Figure 3. Lutiisi Academy Primary School site concept plan with key design elements identified.

Table 2. Lutiisi Academy concept plan element descriptions and benefits.

Table 2. Lutiisi Academy concept plan element descriptions and benefits

Design Element Number & Description	Potential Social, Health & Educational Benefits
1. The Sports Field: Provides activity space for school sporting teams, physical education instruction, health and motor skill development, and community sports and recreation.	• Increased in school attendance. • Increased student health and fitness Increased community health and fitness Increased school pride through sporting team representation. • Increased community socialization through sport and recreation with other communities.
2. New Toilets and Change Rooms: Provides sanitary facilities for staff and children during school hours, and for community members using the school facilities during after school hours.	• Improved school sanitation and hygiene for students, teachers and community members. • Reduction in student and teacher absenteeism due to improved teaching, learning, and overall working conditions.
3. The Lunch Shelter: Provides shelter from rain and sun during lunch and a place for children to sit and talk when not playing or in class.	• Allows children to eat lunch and talk together outside of the classroom, even during hot or rainy weather. • Provides a covered outdoor classroom space for teachers teaching agriculture and science to students. • Allows the community a place to sit and watch when using the sporting field or play spaces at the school.
4. School Solar Energy Panels and Solar Hot Water System: Provides electrical energy for water pumps, lighting, computers and other instructional technologies, as well as potable water and clean water for hygiene and sanitation use.	• Increased opportunities for teacher and community professional development. • Increased opportunities for student technology experiences and education. • Increased opportunities for alternative educational teaching methodologies. • Improved education and teaching quality, student attendance and educational performance scores. • Cleaner water and hot water for washing. • Teacher housing power and drinking water. • Reduction in teacher and student absenteeism due to improved health learning and working conditions.
5. K Through P2 Playground: Provides age appropriate activity and play space for children in Grades K through P2.	• Increased early motor skill development opportunities for preschool through P2 age children. • Increased health and movement opportunities and experiences for young children. • Increased student enrollment and attendance in school.
6. P3 Through P7 Playground: Provides age appropriate activity and play space for children in Grades P3 through P7.	• Increased age appropriate motor skill development opportunities for children in P3 through P7 classes. • Increased health and movement opportunities and experiences for young children. • Increased student enrollment and attendance in school.

Design Element Number & Description	Potential Social, Health & Educational Benefits
7. Visitor Parking: Provides an area for those visiting the school to park their cars off the school property.	• Increased student safety. • Increased parking opportunities for other schools and communities who are visiting the school to participate in programs and sports.
8. School Courtyard Garden and Flagpole: Provides a garden and sitting area for teachers and students in the school courtyard, and a place for the national flag in front of the school.	• Increased aquifer recharge, water retention and containment of roof runoff water that pools in the courtyard. • Increased aesthetic quality of the school • Increased biology educational opportunities if used as an outdoor education area
9. The Nandi Tree: Provides color and aesthetic to the school site, shade for children in the lunch area, soil stability, aquifer recharge, and a landmark feature for identifying the school.	• Increased rain cover and shade area for the children during lunchtime. • Increased soil stability and aquifer recharge • Increased school recognition and identification due to the size of this tree and the readily recognizable red flower it produces.
10. The Cassia Tree: Provides color and aesthetic to the school site, shade for children in the play area, soil stability, aquifer recharge, and a landmark feature for identifying the school.	• Increased rain-cover and shade area for the children playing in the K through P2 play area. • Increased soil stability and aquifer recharge • Increased school recognition and identification due to the readily recognizable yellow flower it produces.
11. Wild Magnolia Tree-lined School Entranceway: Provides a well-defined and attractive entranceway to the school building.	• Increases the aesthetic quality and attractiveness of the school • Increases the recognition of the school and provides a landmark and identifiable entranceway to the school for students and community members.
12. Three-sister Permaculture Agriculture Instructional Area: Provides an area for both students and community members wishing to learn more about permaculture as an agricultural method.	• Increased educational opportunities for students and community members to learn about permaculture and environmentally sustainable agricultural food production strategies. • Increased food production for use at the school.
13. Four 5,000 Liter Water Storage Tanks: Provides additional water storage for use by students, teachers, the community, and for agriculture.	• Increased amounts of water that can now be used for drinking, hygiene, sanitation, and cooking – all leading to the increased health of the teachers and students. • Increased educational opportunities to teach hygienic practices related to cleaning and sanitation. • Increased guarantee of water supply during drought prone periods allows for educational opportunities like raising livestock for both students and the community. This in turn increases food production for the school, variety and type of food produced at the school, and the health of the students and teachers there.

Table 2. (Continued)

Design Element Number & Description	Potential Social, Health & Educational Benefits
14. School Side Garden: Provides color and aesthetic to the school site, aquifer recharge, and soil stability in a drainage swale that runs alongside the school.	• Increased water capture and aquifer recharge and an overall reduction in topsoil runoff during periods of high rainfall. • Increased aesthetic for the school. • Ideal food source for bees as a potential small business opportunity for the school and community. • Increased educational opportunities as an outdoor learning environment for students in the area of sustainability, environmental protection, and plant biology.
15. Assorted Native Flowering and Fruit Trees: Provides food, shade, and flowers for the school while helping to reduce topsoil erosion and site water runoff.	• Increased access to food/fruit sources for the school students and teachers. • Increased food source for the community and as a potential small business opportunity. • Ideal food source for bees and honey production as a small business opportunity. • Increased shade around the sport fields for student, teacher, and community spectators. • Increased soil stability and aquifer recharge, as well as reduced levels of water runoff from the school site onto neighboring properties.
16. School Orchard: Provides food for the school, educational opportunities in agriculture, small business opportunities for the school and surrounding community, as well as a safe environment to keep bees and an apiary.	• Increased access to fresh food for the school-teachers and students. • Increased educational opportunities for students and community members in agriculture and biology. • Accentuates views from teacher housing. • Source of compost and food for livestock. • Increased small business opportunities for both the school and community members as a result of additional food/fruit production and honey production from apiary.
17. Teacher Housing: Provides on-site accommodation for teachers working at the school.	• Increased appeal of school for teacher recruitment. • Reduced teacher absenteeism and attrition. • Increased security for the school, livestock, and other agricultural areas of the school during periods when students are not in school. • Allows for onsite care of livestock by teachers during periods when students are not in school. • Reduced teacher travel costs to school. • Increased job and life stability for teachers. • Increased opportunity to collect potable water from roof runoff. • Increased source for solar hot water and electrical energy production for use by teachers.

Design Element Number & Description	Potential Social, Health & Educational Benefits
18. Shelters and Water Storage Tanks for School Livestock: Provides enclosed and sheltered areas to raise small livestock (e.g., chickens, rabbits, etc.), adding to the agricultural curriculum currently provided to students by the school.	• Additional food sources for students, teachers and community members. • Increased educational opportunities for students and community members in agriculture and livestock husbandry and care. • Increased small business opportunities for the school and community based on products resulting from livestock as a food source. • Provides a source of compost and fertilizer for use in other agricultural areas in the school.
19. Open Livestock Pens: Provides a safe and contained movement area for the raising of larger livestock (e.g., goats).	• Additional food sources for students, teachers and community members. • Increased educational opportunities for students and community members in agriculture and livestock husbandry and care. • Increased small business opportunities for the school and community based on products resulting from livestock as a food source. • Provides a source of compost and fertilizer for use in other agricultural areas in the school.
20. School Honey Production Microenterprise Area: Provides honey production for both school food use and for sale, and while supporting fruit development through bee pollination of the school orchard and surrounding fruit trees.	• Additional food source for the school teachers and students. • Additional income for the school through the sale of honey as a community supported small business microenterprise • Increased educational opportunities in small business, agriculture and food productions sciences. • Increased community support and involvement in the school through the management of the school's honey production microenterprise.
21. Teacher Gardens: Provides areas for teachers to grow vegetables, flowers, and keep animals for personal use and food supplementation.	• Additional source of food for teachers and a reduced cost of living in terms of food expenses. • Increased life and job stability. • Increased teacher recruitment potential and reduced teacher absence and attrition. • Improved school appeal as an employer for teachers.
22. School Southside Agricultural Field: Provides food for students and teachers at the school as well as educational opportunities for students in agriculture.	• Increased food opportunities for students and teachers at the school. • Increased educational opportunities in the areas of science education, agricultural education, and environmental education. • Additional food source for livestock and potential compost for agriculture.

Table 2. (Continued)

Design Element Number & Description	Potential Social, Health & Educational Benefits
23. Apiary: Provides honey for student consumption and school or community business microenterprise.	• Low cost, low maintenance source of food and income for the school and community. • Additional revenue source for the school. • Increased educational opportunities in biology, environmental and agricultural education for both students at the school and community members. • Increased opportunities for school and student community service involvement.
24. New School Kitchen and Shop: Provides cooking facilities for teacher and student lunches as well as an outlet for the sale of school supplies to students.	• Addition of the kitchen roof as a source for energy collection, water collection, and water treatment through the use of solar energy panels and solar hot water systems. • Increased amounts of potable water for drinking and safe water for cooking and hygiene activities for students and teachers. • Increased availability of electricity through renewable energy sources.
25. Assorted Native Flowering and Fruit Trees: Provides food, shade, and flowers for the teacher housing area while helping to reduce topsoil erosion and site water runoff.	• Increased food availability for teachers supplementing their income by growing and harvesting from local native food sources for themselves. • Increased food source for the community and as a potential small business opportunity. • Increased school aesthetic and appeal for teachers seeking employment. • Ideal food source for bees and honey production as a small business opportunity. • Increased natural shade around the teacher housing area. • Increased soil stability and aquifer recharge, as well as reduced levels of water runoff and potential topsoil erosion onto the school's south side agricultural field.
26. Living Fences from Hedges, Berry Shrubs and Vines: Provides food as well as fencing to prevent animals from neighboring properties from grazing on school property or on crops being grown at the school.	• Additional source of food for school students, teachers, and community members. • Improved visual aesthetics for the school. • Reduction in crop/food loss due to neighboring farm animal incursions. • Increased safety for students through fewer animal incursions into the school property.

A series of 24 inch by 36 inch posters were created displaying the children's artwork, site analysis, results of the data collection process, site concept plan, and associated site sections and perspectives. These posters were taken to the Lutiisi Academy primary school by the BT Foundation staff and shown to the students, teachers, School Management Committee, and community members who had participated in the site concept plan development. These participants reviewed the posters, discussed changes and revisions they thought important, and considered the feasibility of implementing these design ideas at the Lutiisi Academy primary school.

Discussion

An initial site concept plan, along with images depicting what that plan might look like, was developed based on the information, activities, and conversations with the school students, teachers, School Management Committee, and community members. These plans were presented back to the participant groups so that they could envision the Lutiisi Academy primary school as more than just a building with classrooms. While some of the elements in the site concept plan, like the sporting fields, require significant capital outlay and engineering of the site, other elements like the creation of the school food gardens and orchard, would be relatively easy to create. These elements would only need the seeds or cuttings, and some human effort, to become a reality. Indeed, site concept plan elements like the school gardens could even be created by the students at the school, and infused into a science or community service lesson by their teacher. Overall, it was envisioned that these images would act as a catalyst for discussion and provide students, teachers, the School Management Committee, and community members with some potential areas in which they could initiate change.

The community-centered design process accomplished these goals. The initial conversations and resulting plans stimulated further discussion and ideas regarding the school's landscape. This allowed the group to explore other options in addition to those offered in the site concept plan. For example, the provision of teacher housing at the southern end of the site was of particular interest to the teachers, School Management Committee, and community members. Each of these participant groups had indicated that teacher housing should be located at the school. The inclusion of teacher housing would help address issues like teacher absenteeism and turnover rates in rural areas (24–26), and may even act as an employment incentive for good teachers to come and work at the Lutiisi Academy primary school. However, these participant groups did not think the provision of separate housing units, as displayed in the site concept plan, were necessary or feasible. While the location of the teacher housing was thought to be appropriate, the teachers, School Management Committee, and community members concluded that townhouse style accommodation (i.e., a series of apartment style homes in one large building with common dividing walls separating each home) would be more appropriate and feasible to develop financially.

Construction has now begun on the townhouse style teacher housing at the Lutiisi Academy primary school in the area proposed on the site concept plan. Further, this teacher housing construction is being completed by the Lutiisi Academy primary school community members themselves, without support or help from BT or other outside organizations (see Figure 4). At the heart of this process is the concept that design can act as a catalyst for change and that this change is most likely when community members actively participate in the process and are empowered as decision makers. As Schuman (2006) notes, neighborhood participation in the design and planning process reflects:

> "a growing recognition that neighborhood involvement produces better plans. It engenders local "ownership" of the plan that can foster long-term stewardship of public

spaces. And, it values local residents as assets for their skills and knowledge. As a practical matter, community endorsement means a smoother road to implementation (27)."

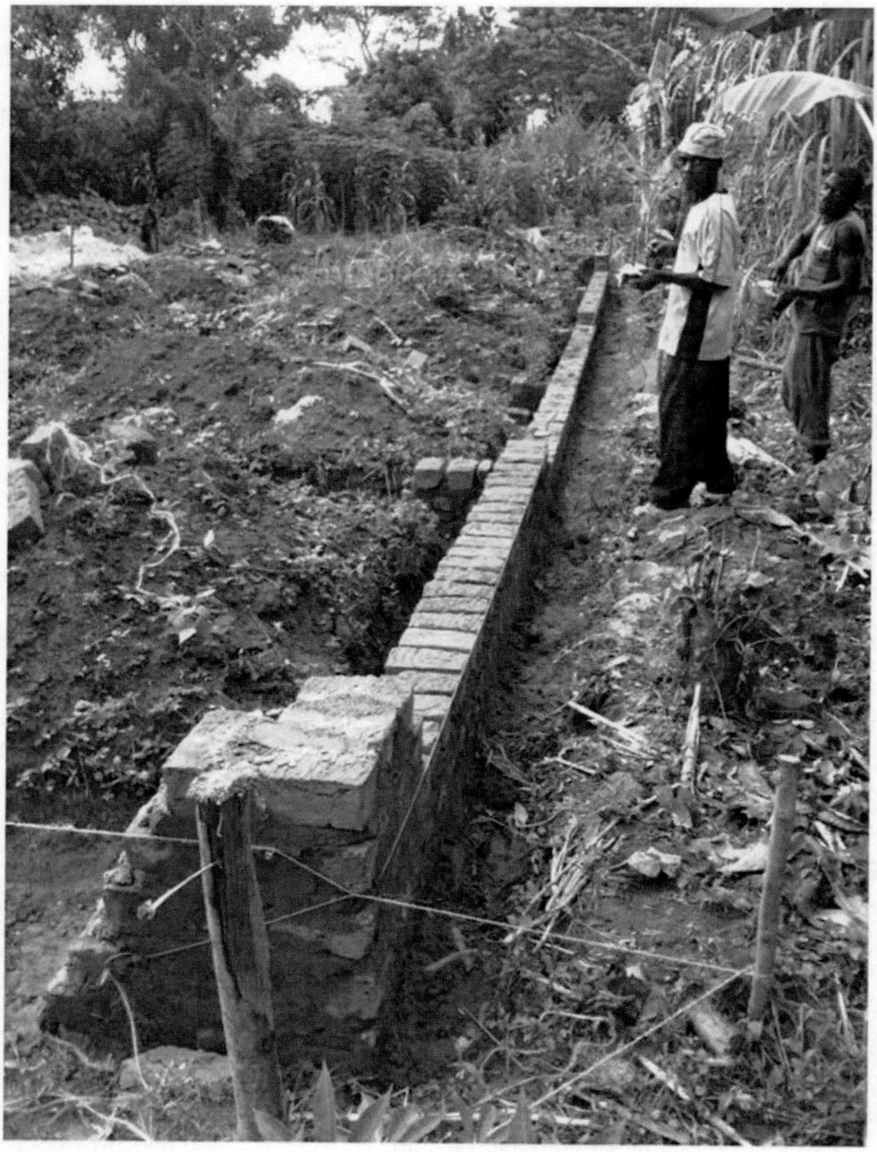

Figure 4. Lutiisi Academy Primary School teacher housing foundations being built.

Acknowledgments

Our thanks to Dr Najma Dahrani at the Kenyatta University School of Environmental Studies for her assistance in the identification of native vegetation, farming, and permaculture practices in East Central Africa. Additional thanks must go to Mr. George Srour, Mr. Joseph Kaliisa, Mr. William Kajubi, and the staff of Building Tomorrow in both the United States and Uganda. This project would not have been possible without the logistical support of this organization and the on-going assistance of these individuals. Finally, I would like to express my appreciation and thanks to the principal, teachers, students, School Management Committee, and community members of the Lutiisi Academy Primary School in Wakiso, Uganda. Their thoughts, voices, and actions are the essence of this study and I wish them success as they continue to create opportunities that improve their lives, and the lives of their children at the school.

References

[1] Grogan L. Universal primary education and school entry in Uganda. J Afr Econ 2009;18(2):183–211.

[2] United Nations General Assembly UN. Millenium Report of the Secretary-General of the United Nations [Internet]. Assembly UNG, ed. United Nations Website; 2000. URL: http://www.un.org/millennium/sg/report/index.html

[3] Juuko FW, Kabonesa C. Universal primary education (UPE) in contemporary Uganda: right or priveledge? HURIPEC Working Paper 2007;8:55. URL; www.huripec.mak.ac.ug/working_paper_8.pdf

[4] Nakabugo MG, Byamugisha A, Bithaghalire J. Future schooling in Uganda. J Int Coop Educ 2008;11(1):55–69.

[5] Ministry for Education and Sports (MoES). A comprehensive analysis of basic education in Uganda. Ministry for Education and Sports (MoES), ed. Kampala, Uganda: Ministry Education Sports, 2005.

[6] Chabbott C. UNICEFs child friendly schools: Case study Uganda. Child Friendly Schools. UNICEF, 2010.

[7] Srour G. Building tomorrow, 2014. URL: www.buildingtomorrow.org

[8] The Republic of Uganda Ministry of Education and Sports. Primary Seven Curriculum. Sports R of UM of E, ed. Kampala, Uganda: National Curriculum Development Center, 2012.

[9] Mucunguzi P. Environmental education in the formal sector of education in Uganda. Environ Educ Res 1995;1(2):233.

[10] Muyanda-Mutebi P. An analysis of the primary education curriculum in Uganda including a framework for a primary education curriculum renewal. Nairobi, Kenya: ASESP, 1996:47.

[11] Blair D. The child in the garden: An evaluative review of the benefits of school gardening. J Environ Educ 2009;40(2):15–38.

[12] Thompson CW, Aspinall P, Montarizino A. The childhood factor: Adult visits to green places and the significance of childhood experience. Environ Behav 2008;40(1):111–43.

[13] Moore RC, Cooper Marcus C. The importance of designing spaces that support children's contact with nature. In: Keller S, Heerwagen J, Mador M, eds. Biohpic design: Theory, science and practice. Hoboken, NJ: John Wiley, 2008.

[14] Wells NM, Lekies K. Nature and the life course: Pathways from childhood nature experiences to adult environmentalism. Child Youth Environ 2006;16(1):1–24.

[15] Trudeau F, Shephard RJ. Physical education, school physical activity, school sports and academic performance. Int J Behav Nutr Phys Act 2008;5:10.

[16] Rowe PG. Design thinking. Boston, MA: MIT Press, 1987.

[17] Motloch J. Introduction to landscape design, 2nd ed. New York: John Wiley, 2001.

[18] Dillon J, Rickinson M, Teamey K, Morris M, Choi MY, Sanders D, et al. The value of outdoor learning: Evidence from research in the UK and elsewhere. Sch Sci Rev 2006;87:107–11.

[19] Minkler M, Wallerstein N. Community based participatory research for health; From process to outcome. San Fransisco, CA: Jossey-Bass, 2008.

[20] Woolner P, Clark J, Hall E, Tiplady L, Thomas U, Wall K. Pictures are necessary but not sufficient: Using a range of visual methods to engage users about school design. Learn Environ Res 2010;13(1):1–22.

[21] Woolner P, Hall E, Wall K, Dennison D. Getting together to improve the school environment: User consultation, participatory design and student voice. Improv Sch 2007;10(3):233–48.

[22] Carlson M. Kids know their school best. Educ Facil Plan 2010;44(4):13–6.

[23] McNaught C, Lam P. Using wordle as a supplementary research tool. Qual Rep 2010;15(3):630–43.

[24] Shiotani A, Barber M, Vermeersch C. Teacher absenteeism and teacher accountability. USAID Educ Startegy Dev 2009;2(6410):1–10.

[25] Chaudhury N, Hammer J, Kremer M, Muralidharan K, Rogers FH. Missing in action. Teacher Health 2006;20(1):91–116.

[26] Ariba C. Uganda: Teacher absenteeism in Teso stands at 50 percent. New Vision 2013 May 01. URL: http://allafrica.com/stories/201305010681.html

[27] Schuman AW. The Pedogogy of Engagement. In: Hardin MC, Eribes R, Poster C, eds. From the studio to the streets. Sterling, VA: Stylus, 2006.

In: Public Health
Editors: Rosemary M. Caron and Joav Merrick

ISBN: 978-1-63321-569-6

Chapter 15

Building a co-created citizen science program with gardeners neighboring a superfund site: The Gardenroots case study

Monica D Ramirez-Andreotta, MPA, PhD*[1*]*,
Mark L Brusseau, PhD*[1,2]*, Janick F Artiola, PhD*[1]*,
***Raina M Maier, PhD*[1] *and A Jay Gandolfi, PhD*[3]**
[1] Department of Soil, Water and Environmental Science
[2] Department of Hydrology and Water Resources Department
[3] Department of Pharmacology and Toxicology, The University of Arizona, Tucson, Arizona, US

A research project that is only expert-driven may ignore the role of local knowledge in research, give low priority to the development of a comprehensive communication strategy to engage the community, and may not deliver the results of the study to the community in an effective way. Objective: To demonstrate how a research program can respond to a community research need, establish a community-academic partnership, and build a co-created citizen science program. Methods: A place-based, community-driven project was designed where academics and community members maintained a reciprocal dialogue, and together, we: 1) defined the question for study, 2) gathered information, 3) developed hypotheses, 3) designed data collection methodologies, 4) collected environmental samples (soil, irrigation water, and vegetables), 5) interpreted data, 6) disseminated results and translated results into action, and 7) discussed results and asked new questions. Results: The co-created environmental research project produced new data and addressed an additional exposure route (consumption of vegetables grown in soils with elevated arsenic levels). Public participation in scientific research improved

* Correspondence*:* Assistant Professor Monica D Ramirez-Andreotta, MPA, PhD, Department of Health Sciences, Bouvé College of Health Sciences Northeastern University, 360 Huntington Avenue, 336INV, Boston, MA 02115, United States. E-mail: m.ramirezandreotta@neu.edu.

environmental health assessment, information transfer, and risk communication efforts. Furthermore, incorporating the community in the scientific process produced both individual learning outcomes and community-level outcomes. Conclusions: This approach illustrates the benefits of a community-academic co-created citizen-science program in addressing the complex problems that arise in communities neighboring a contaminated site. Such a project can increase the community's involvement in risk communication and decision-making, which ultimately has the potential to help mitigate exposure and thereby reduce associated risk.

List of acronyms

USEPA	US Environmental Protection Agency
NPL	National Priorities List
CBPR	Community based participatory research
PPSR	Public participation in scientific research
UASRP-RTC	University of Arizona Superfund Research Program Research Translation Coordinator
NIEHS	National Institute of Environmental Health Sciences
UA	The University of Arizona
ADEQ	Arizona Department of Environmental Quality
Iron King	Iron King Mine and Humboldt Smelter Superfund Site

Introduction

Typically community members living in contaminated communities are the ones who initially identify adverse ecological and health outcomes associated with toxic exposures (1), although a state agency, regional US Environmental Protection Agency (USEPA) office, or the responsible party may also make this discovery. The USEPA may add the site to the Comprehensive Environmental Response, Compensation, and Liability Information System, which can lead to a cascade of regulatory and/or remedy events. For example, sites on the National Priorities List (NPL) with groundwater contamination, the time from discovery to remedy implementation can go beyond 20 years, and long-term management (i.e. decades to centuries) is needed at many sites (2). As time passes, site managers are responsible for monitoring the progress of remediation and engaging the community to inform them of the cleanup progress and describe potential risks associated with the site.

Traditionally, site managers engage the community in a one-way communication model that solely aims to inform, change behavior, and assure populations that the determined risk is acceptable and that cleanup is underway (3, 4). This communication strategy has a low rate of success, primarily because it excludes those most affected (3) and fundamentally does not aim to increase environmental education or involve the community in the decisions about their risk. Historically, because communities were not involved in the decision-making process, mistrust often eroded the relationships between scientists, regulatory officials, and the affected communities (5,6).

The lack of public participation at contaminated sites is a great loss, as community members have been contributing to science since the 17th century (7, 8) and in general, volunteerism is considered critical to civic life in the United States (9,10). Volunteers have monitored watershed health in more than 700 programs in the US, involving over 400,000 local stakeholders (11) and most ecological research once fostered public participation in most or all of the steps in the scientific process (8). However, due to the professionalization of science, the role of the amateur scientist has diminished (8). The value of public participation in addressing environmental and health issues has received renewed attention in the past couple of decades through efforts such as public participation in scientific research (PPSR)/ citizen science (12), community based participatory research (CBPR) (13), popular epidemiology (14), and street science (15).

Public participation in scientific research, often termed citizen science, is a form of informal science education, and is broadly defined as a partnership between scientists and non-scientists in which authentic data are collected, shared, and analyzed (12,16,17). Citizen science projects are meant to increase a participant's scientific literacy (12), to collect field data to monitor a variety of environmental conditions (7), and as a framework to support and enhance decision-making in modern society (17,18). Previous research in science education and sociology has demonstrated the need to engage communities in scientific research and that this level of engagement can be successfully facilitated via community-academic partnerships. Members of a community neighboring a contaminated site are typically intrinsically motivated to learn more about the site and in most cases, have already begun to gather additional scientific data and hypothesize other potential routes of exposure and areas that need additional monitoring. Research related to inquiry-based education has elucidated how people have a greater motivation to engage and learn when the subject matter is directly related to their lives and if the learning process is interactive (19). Popular epidemiology, a community-driven practice, was proposed after observing the activities of communities experiencing contamination and entails community initiation of investigations, gathering of scientific knowledge, and, if necessary, recruiting of scientific professionals (14). "Street Science" is an approach for environmental health justice that joins local knowledge with professional techniques, re-values forms of knowledge that professional science has traditionally excluded (15).

To date, only a limited number of co-created PPSR projects, which are jointly developed by members of the public and scientists and designed to actively involve community members in most or all steps of the scientific process, have been initiated at contaminated sites and none in conjunction with risk communication as described herein. This paper will outline the methods and activities employed to build a community-academic partnership that resulted in the co-created citizen science project entitled *Gardenroots: The Dewey-Humboldt, Arizona Garden Project* (hereafter, *Gardenroots*). In order to foster PPSR, it is essential to establish a community–academic partnership via a CBPR approach to research, which shares power with community partners in all aspects of the research process and benefits communities via interventions and policy change (13).

The enhanced CBPR approach presented herein is based upon the belief that PPSR in conjunction with CBPR can improve site assessment and risk communication efforts. Public participation can be a vehicle to address concerns regarding environmental contaminants and exposure routes that might not be addressed in a typical expert-only-led site and risk assessment. Lastly, PPSR provides a unique opportunity for informal science education and a way in which for the community may learn more about environmental science, human health research, and risk assessment.

Methods

The *Gardenroots* approach followed recommended CBPR practices (13). The co-created citizen science project will be described in terms of PPSR (see table 1), demonstrating community involvement in most phases of the research (12). The traditional CBPR/PPSR steps have been enhanced and the methods described herein also include: building a transdisciplinary team, bidirectional communication with government agencies, an informal science education learning continuum, and a substantial risk communication component. Lastly, this project received Institutional Review Board approval.

Background

Gardening and consuming edible plants grown in contaminated soils presents a health hazard that may effect home gardeners neighboring contaminated environments. The town of Dewey-Humboldt is in an arsenic endemic region of Arizona and is adjacent to the Iron King Mine and Humboldt Smelter Superfund site (Iron King). The site serves as a persistent source of pollution, introducing a host of potential human-health risks and concomitant risk communication challenges. Such contamination (natural or human-made) can affect humans directly via the inadvertent consumption of soils, through the consumption of crops grown under contaminated conditions, and/or the consumption of contaminated water.

How a research program can respond to a community research need

Beginning in 2007, the University of Arizona (UA) Superfund Research Program Research Translation Coordinator (UASRP-RTC) and the USEPA Region 9 Superfund and Technology Liaison began executing a two-pronged communication mechanism consisting of a webinar hosted by National Institute of Environmental Sciences (NIEHS) and USEPA and a "Live at R9" in-person seminar to foster regional partnerships (20). During a "Live at R9" visit in June of 2007, an USEPA project manager mentioned that an abandoned mining site located in rural Arizona would be added to the NPL and that UA and EPA might be able to assist in some capacity at the site. The USEPA kept the UASRP-RTC up-to-date on the status of the site and on August 3, 2008 the Iron King Mine Superfund site was listed on the NPL. On August 20, 2008, the USEPA organized their first community "Kick-Off Meeting" after the official listing to discuss the Superfund process and that they were initiating the field investigation portion of the Remedial Investigation and Feasibility Study. Forty-six community members, two members of UASRP-RTC, the USEPA Project Manager and Community Involvement Coordinator, a member of the Arizona Department of Environmental Quality, and the Dewey-Humboldt mayor attended the meeting. During the meeting, several community members asked whether the site has impacted their soil and if they may continue to grown vegetables.

At the end of the meeting, members of the Dewey-Humboldt, community specifically asked the UASRP-RTC "Is it safe to garden and consume vegetables from my home garden? And if so, how much can I eat from my garden?" Without any specific data to conclusively answer the question, a representative of the UASRP-RTC, stated that she was interested in this research question as well, and whether they (the people who expressed concern) were interested in participating in a research project. Residents agreed and in less than two years an academic-community partnership came into fruition that took the form of a co-created citizen science project, *Gardenroots*. The goals of the *Gardenroots* project were to bring scientists from various disciplines together within the UA and to work in collaboration with the affected community to: (1) determine the uptake of arsenic in garden vegetables grown by the Dewey-Humboldt, AZ community, and (2) conduct an exposure assessment and characterize the potential risk posed by gardening and consuming vegetables from residential home gardens.

Establishing a community academic partnership

The community members who originally posed the research question and the lead UA investigator became the point of contact and "champions" (21) for the research project within their affiliations. They were persistent, promoted the project, and networked to obtain the involvement of a broader representation of residents in the area. In addition, the UA investigator made a point to maintain a consistent presence in the community by attending town council, USEPA meetings and community events and was in the area at a minimum frequency of once every two months throughout the duration of *Gardenroots*. It was this type of promotion and dedication that truly fused and generated the community-academic partnership. In addition to promotion, continuity is crucial. To date, the RTC continues to maintain bidirectional communication between the community, EPA, Arizona Department of Environmental Quality (ADEQ), Arizona Department of Health Services, and Agency for Toxic Substances and Disease Registry, via teleconferences and meetings to ensure transparency and unified messaging to the community.

Building a research team

A transdisciplinary team was created involving the Dewey-Humboldt community and the UA including researchers in the disciplines of environmental chemistry and microbiology, soils, hydrology, public health, and visual communications. The UA Cooperative Extension Director of Yavapai County was recruited as part of the team to provide home gardening expertise. Interactions with USEPA Region 9 representatives were ongoing to ensure that this research question was aligned with their current research challenges at the Iron King site.

Building a co-created citizen science research program: public participation in environmental research

As stated above, the UA Investigator maintained a consistent presence in the community by attending town council, USEPA and community meetings and events and was frequently in the Dewey–Humboldt area. Through the continuity of community engagement, the UA investigator built trust and learned a great deal about the nuances and idiosyncrasies of the area. This knowledge facilitated implementation of a place-based communication strategy (22) to recruit other community members into *Gardenroots*. The recruitment and design of recruitment and educational materials was informed by the social context and community ecology of Dewey-Humboldt, Arizona. The majority of the recruitment for *Gardenroots* was done via personal interaction at local community events through the following activities:

- Handing out informational bookmarks (Figure 1) at community festivals, EPA community meetings, and Town Council meetings.
- Follow-up mailings, telephone calls and emails to community members
- A County Cooperative Extension Press Release
- An announcement in the Dewey-Humboldt town newsletter
- A website

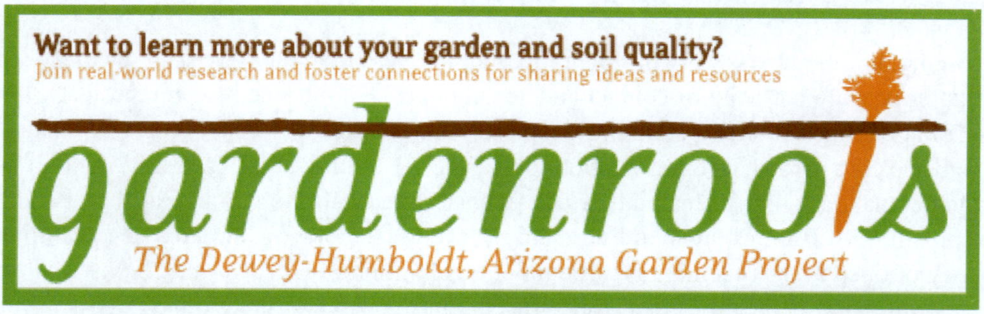
Want to learn more about your garden and soil quality?
Join real-world research and foster connections for sharing ideas and resources
gardenroots
The Dewey-Humboldt, Arizona Garden Project

Front of bookmark

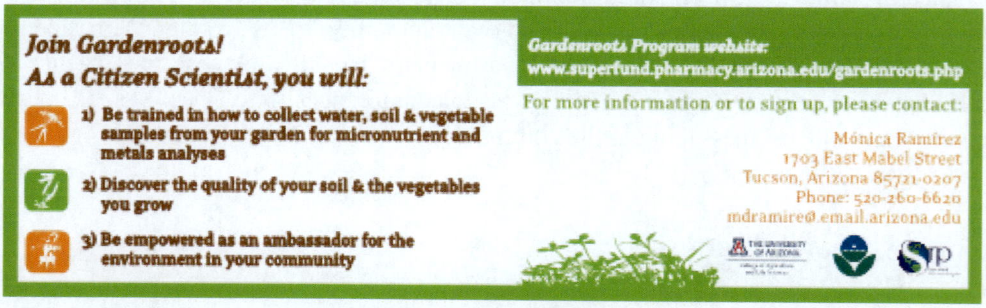
Join Gardenroots!
As a Citizen Scientist, you will:
1) Be trained in how to collect water, soil & vegetable samples from your garden for micronutrient and metals analyses
2) Discover the quality of your soil & the vegetables you grow
3) Be empowered as an ambassador for the environment in your community
Gardenroots Program website:
www.superfund.pharmacy.arizona.edu/gardenroots.php
For more information or to sign up, please contact:
Mónica Ramírez
1703 East Mabel Street
Tucson, Arizona 85721-0207
Phone: 520-260-6620
mdramire@email.arizona.edu

Back of bookmark

Figure 1. Front and back of promotional bookmark distributed at community events to recruit gardeners.

Greenhouse study

Collecting soils from a residential area in Dewey-Humboldt, AZ was fundamental to conducting the controlled greenhouse study. Since the USEPA had already begun the site investigation, members of the community had been given their residential soil results. Based on their results, a community member offered their soils for the greenhouse study and assisted in identifying the appropriate locations to collect soils in their yard based upon the USEPA data and their understanding of the neighboring watershed. In addition, this community member provided detailed historical information regarding their property and areas of interest realted to the Iron King site.

Field study

After all recruitment activities discussed above were completed, those who signed up for *Gardenroots* were asked to attend a 1.5-hour training session wherein they were provided information on how to properly collect soil, water, and vegetables samples from their home garden for laboratory analysis. Two trainings were formally offered and community members that participated in the training took home an instructional manual (Figure 2A) and a tool kit with all supplies required for sample collection from their home garden. Several community members were unable to attend a scheduled training. An additional less formal training was offered and in some instances, kits were personally delivered to community member's homes at their request.

During the five-month period from when participants received their kit and during the Spring/Summer growing season, participants were asked to deliver their samples to the local Cooperative Extension office. The in-person training, designing a user-friendly manual, and collaborating with the local extension office assured sample quality. In the end, participants actively contributed to the field study portion of *Gardenroots*. Table 1 outlines the steps in scientific research, level of public participation, the community's role and benefits, and challenges associated with each step.

Capacity building and continuity

In order to properly and effectively manage community expectation and involvement throughout the entire *Gardenroots* project (from the posing of the research question to the final community report-back events), ongoing communication was maintained via phone, email and mail correspondence, and informal science education experiences were offered. Based upon what the community wanted to learn, and in efforts to further understand their concerns regarding the Iron King site, the *Gardenroots* Learning Continuum was designed to provide participants with responsive, unique, and informal learning opportunities (Figure 2) throughout the course of the *Gardenroots* project. *Gardenroots* culminated in a large report-back gathering "Results for Lunch: Your Soil, Water and Vegetable Outcomes" (Results for Lunch). After the Results for Lunch gathering (Figure 2B), participants requested an overall summary of results and presentations that would be open to the broader community.

Table 1. The components of *Gardenroots*: The Dewey-Humboldt, Arizona Garden Project

Steps in Scientific Research	Participant Participation	Community Roles and Benefits	Challenges Associated with Step
Choose or define question(s) for study	√	• Community members posed research question at the EPA Superfund Site Kick Off Meeting in August 2008	• It took a year to secure funding for the project
Gather information and resources	√	• Community member provided soils for greenhouse study • Yavapai and Pima County Master Gardeners in the area assisted with what to grown in the greenhouse. • Participants were asked to describe how he or she amends their soils.	• Reaching all community members in the area interested in vegetable gardening

Develop explanations (hypotheses)	√	• At trainings, community members developed hypotheses regarding what they expected to observe in their household results and for the entire study.
		    ○ For example, several participants hypothesized that the closer to the tailings a home was, the higher the arsenic concentration would be in the soils.
			• Setting and maintaining expectations. It was important to restate goals and what type of data could truly be expected from *Gardenroots*.
			• Explaining that the number of samples was not sufficient to truly characterize the spatial distribution of arsenic as well as the complexity and uncertainty related to the atmospheric distribution of arsenic.
			    ○ For example, wind direction in the area changes seasonally, the area has naturally occurring arsenic and has been affected by both smelting and mine tailings, which produce different sized particles that can experience different levels of transport by wind.

Design data collection methodologies	√	• Participants decided where to collect soils from their residential property (garden and yard) and what vegetables they wanted analyzed	• Since there was not one predetermined vegetable grown in every garden, it was challenging to compare across households. Regardless, it was important to have participants grow what they wanted to make sure the study was relevant and applicable to everyone. • Explaining that the one area they sampled might not be representative of their entire yard and that arsenic soil concentrations may vary in a relatively small spatial area.

Steps in Scientific Research	**Participant Participation**	Community Roles and Benefits	Challenges Associated with Step
Collect samples and/or record data	√	• Participants collected their soil, vegetable and irrigation samples • Participants labeled all samples	• No major challenges to report.
Analyze samples	X	• Community did not participate in this step, although at community gatherings, analytical methodology was described in great detail	• Due to the nature of the sample analyses and formal laboratory procedures, the participants did not get to prepare their samples via acid digestion or analyze samples via inductively coupled plasma mass spectrometry.
Analyze data	X	• Community did not participate in this step, UA investigator analyzed all the data. • At the "Results for Lunch" and other community gatherings, the methods and mathematical equations used to interpret the data was described in great detail and participants were given the opportunity to recalculate their potential exposure and risk and change the variables to suit their behavior.	• No challenges to report.
Interpret data and draw conclusions	√	• Participants were given the results from their individual soil, water, and vegetable samples, exposure assessment and risk characterization results. • At community gatherings and meetings, the aggregated results were presented	• Determining whether their soil and water arsenic concentrations may be due to naturally occurring and/or from anthropogenic sources like the mine and smelter.
Disseminate conclusions/ translate results into action	√	• Participants shared data with others outside of the *Gardenroots* project • Using their data, participants have translated the results into personal action and have modified their gardening practices.	• Even though *Gardenroots* informed and invited USEPA and ADEQ to all report-back and community events, it was challenging to maintain bidirectional communication between the project and all government agencies working at the site.
Discuss results and ask new questions	√	• At the "Results for Lunch" and other community gatherings, results were discussed in detail, participants compared their results to their neighbors and friends and new questions were posed.	• Since *Gardenroots* was an environmental monitoring project, inquiries regarding potential health outcomes were outside the feasibility of *Gardenroots*. In these cases, the expectations and goals of *Gardenroots* were restated and the inquiries were forwarded to health scientists at the UA.

In response, three additional presentations were given and a "Summary of Results" booklet was generated and distributed to participants and other community members in the Dewey-Humboldt, Arizona area. In addition to the *Gardenroots* Learning Continuum, and as stated in the Field Study section above, participants were actively involved in most steps of the scientific process (Table 1) and this high level of participation was instrumental in building capacity and maintaining continuity.

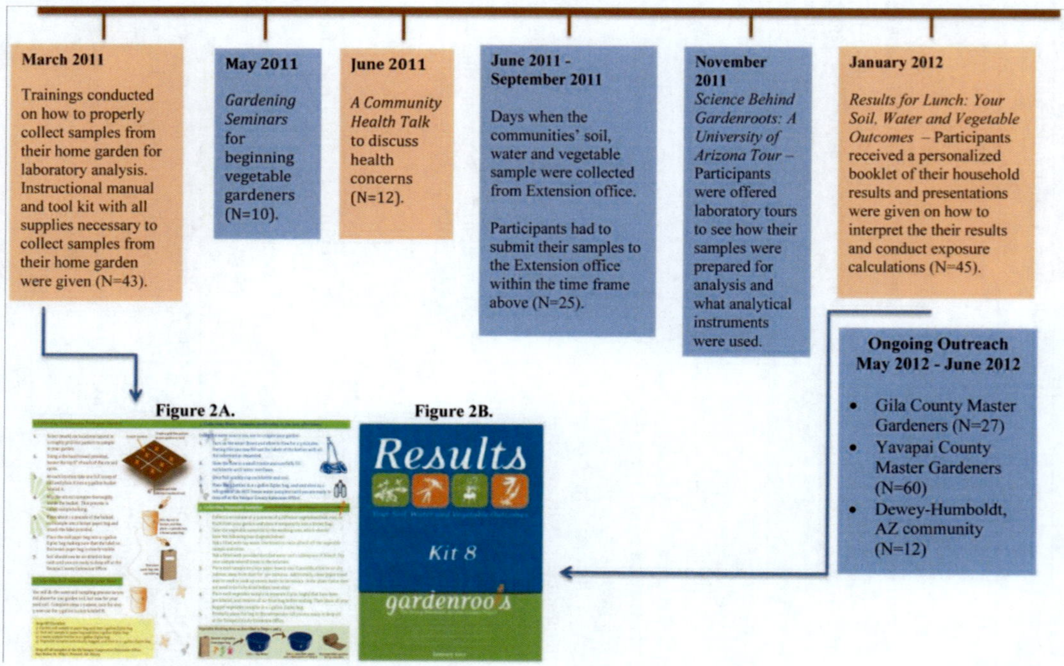

Figure 2. *Gardenroots* Learning Continuum and collection times. The time line demonstrates the activities and co-learning opportunities (N = Number of participants at each event) provided throughout the program.

Risk communication

Once all community samples had been analyzed, results were reported back to the participants to answer questions such as: Can I consume vegetables from my garden? If so, how much is safe? To do this, participants were invited to the Results for Lunch gathering, where they were given an informal presentation on the: 1) methodologies used to prepare and analyze their household samples, 2) exposure assessment and risk characterization calculations used to interpret their data, and 3) an introduction to the format in which their results would be presented. Next, they were given tailored personalized booklets (Figure 2B) that contained the "raw" confidential data (i.e., milligrams of arsenic per kilogram of vegetable) as well as a table that outlined the quantity of vegetables they could consume at various target risk levels compared to the US Department of Agriculture recommended amounts (Supplemental Fig. 1). It is important to emphasize that intake rates based on the site-specific characteristics of their individual garden were calculated for each participant to consider. Additionally, the concentrations observed in the vegetables were compared to the concentrations of arsenic reported in the U.S. Food and Drug Administration Total Diet Study Statistics on Element Results based on the 2006–2008 Market Basket Study. The Market Basket Study involved purchasing samples of food throughout the U.S., preparing the food as it would be consumed, and analyzing the foods to measure the concentrations of selected elements and compounds. This provided a valuable frame of reference and is considered an acceptable risk comparison (5). This reporting method was designed to give participants all the information they requested and allow them to decide for themselves the target risk they wanted to achieve (Table 2).

Table 2. Comparing report-back efforts and what information *Gardenroots* participants were provided throughout the project

Typical participant questions about personal exposure results, Brody et al., 2007	Information provided to *Gardenroots* participants
Description	
What did you find?[1] What did you look for?	Concentration of arsenic (contaminant of concern) and 19 other elements of potential interest
How much?[1]	Concentrations for all 20 elements were presented in a chart for all their vegetables, soil and water samples analyzed.
Analysis/Comparison	
Is that high? [1]	Arsenic concentrations observed in vegetables from the USDFA Market Basket Study were used for comparison. Regional soil screening levels and the maximum contaminant levels in water was provided.
Is that safe?[1]	Chart exhibiting how much of the vegetable can be consumed from their garden at various excess target risks
What should I focus on?	Participants were able to compare the risk posed from each exposure route (water, soil, vegetable) and the arsenic concentration in each vegetable to then decide where to focus mitigation efforts
Where did the chemical come from?	Participants identified their gardens as potential sources of arsenic and initially asked the research question
Recommendation	
What can/should I do?[1]	Exposure reduction/precautionary strategies were provided such as: recommended gardening practices handouts were generated to guide gardeners, "Arizona Know Your Water" and "Arizona Know Your Well Water" guides*

[1]These question were also posed by the Dewey-Humboldt, AZ community in the initial stages and of the study. All report back materials were designed to provide answers to participant's specific questions and coincide with those observed by Brody et al., 2007.

*All handouts and guides were distributed at community gatherings and are available at: and http://www.superfund.pharmacy.arizona.edu/content/informational-materials.

The risk associated with consumption of garden vegetables was also compared to risks associated with other potential exposure routes, such as ingestion of potable water and incidental soil ingestion. It was strongly recommended that home gardeners: sample their private wells regularly, test their soils prior to gardening, and modify their gardening behavior to reduce incidental soil ingestion (23). Based upon these findings, three waterproof handouts were developed to disseminate the recommended behavioral modifications necessary to reduce arsenic exposure from incidental soil ingestion and vegetable consumption (Supplemental Fig. 4, available at http://www.superfund.pharmacy.arizona.edu/content/Gardenroots).

Findings

Forty-three individuals attended the training and received a *Gardenroots* toolkit and instructional manual, 58% or 25 participants actually completed the *Gardenroots* project, and of the participants, 18 completed a survey. Eighty-four percent of the population has some type of education beyond high school, 44% had been living in the area for 8 or more years, and 94% of the participants were Caucasian (Supplemental Table 1). Based on the most recent US Census Bureau, the demographics are reflective of the area, except 28% of the *Gardenroots* participants had a bachelor's degree or higher compared to 13.5% for the general population.

Outcomes

It has been suggested that citizen science learning outcomes can best be evaluated by observing three levels: individual learning, programmatic, and community-level outcomes (24). This is very similar to the evaluation strategies used to report CBPR program successes in the Northern California Household Exposure Study (25) and in 54 National Institute of Environmental Health Sciences funded environmental justice projects (26). Below, we apply this new framework and describe the results and outcomes of the *Gardenroots* project.

Individual learning outcomes – what community members learned and new research questions posed

The results of *Gardenroots* indicated that for the Dewey-Humboldt community mitigating arsenic exposure from potable water and incidental soil ingestion (not even considering vegetable consumption) would significantly reduce daily arsenic intake. The challenge in communicating these results was the fear that the participants, realizing that their water and soil arsenic levels were high, would no longer want to garden or consume vegetables from their garden, regardless of the comparatively low arsenic exposure from their raw vegetables. Fortunately, the majority of the participants stated that they would continue to eat home-garden vegetables, but would modify their gardening practices. This demonstrates that the scientific findings were understood and that the community could put into action behavioral changes necessary to reduce their arsenic exposure from water and soil. This capacity demonstrated by participants is similar to what has been previously reported, where community members demonstrated a capacity to understand and contend with the complexity and uncertainty associated with the results (27).

Analysis of individual learning also showed that *Gardenroots* prompted curiosity and an increased understanding of soil contamination, food quality, and the scientific process.

Several participants asked to have their chicken eggs sampled to determine the concentrations of arsenic and heavy metals. They hypothesized that the deaths of some of their chickens were due to the arsenic and heavy metal concentrations observed in their potable water, soil, and vegetables. Further, they wanted to determine if there was a correlation between the exposure pathways and the concentrations found in the eggs. Another participant inquired whether cinder blocks in a raised garden bed contributed arsenic to their soil, and if samples from the local river or the soil from a local farm had been tested. Participants' questions were answered and the chicken eggs were analyzed. Results were reported back to the participants, who then shared the results with others. These inquiries signify the increase in capacity within the community and could also constitute a community-level outcome.

When comparing report-back methodologies by Brody et al., (2007) and those used for *Gardenroots*, one can observe many similarities in what participants want to know and how to make the information meaningful for action (see table 2). In summary, the UA scientists learned the importance of reporting individual results with an understanding of what people want and need to know to guide action, as witnessed in other studies (29). Additionally, it is important to present specific steps that the community can take to assert some level of control in their lives and methods in which they can implement to reduce their exposure to potential environmental hazards (5).

Programmatic outcomes

The *Gardenroots* project has contributed to the fields of environmental science, environmental health, and research translation. Currently, there is limited information regarding combined arsenic exposure from water, soil, and homegrown vegetables neighboring hazardous waste sites. This PPSR project has improved our understanding of: 1) the uptake of arsenic in common homegrown vegetables grown in soils near a mining site (28); and 2) the amount of arsenic introduced to an individual via the ingestion of homegrown vegetables, soils (incidental), and water, and potential risks posed by those exposure routes (23). This data has been published and demonstrates that community members can successfully participate in environmental science investigations. Lastly, *Gardenroots* participants reviewed this manuscript to ensure the integrity of the project and representation of the partnership.

Community-level outcomes – redefining the question and policy implications

Gardenroots increased social capital and community capacity by serving as a platform for participants to learn more about environmental contamination in general and the Iron King site, and was a catalyst to generate environmental communication efforts amongst the participants and the rest of the community. As a result, participants increased their community networking in resource-related issues and participated in other resource-related projects. Based on conversations with participants, there was interest in leveraging the results to pressure government officials to take action and be more stringent in their cleanup efforts. This is similar to other work in contaminated areas (27).

For example, the *Gardenroots* project revealed that the local public water system was serving water that exceeded the arsenic drinking water standard (0.010 mg/L). *Gardenroots* participants worked together to identify and notify additional households that were connected to the public water supply. They also reported their test results to USEPA and ADEQ, advocating that this issue needed to be addressed (UA also notified and sent the results to the USEPA). As a result, the municipal water suppler was issued seven Notices of Violation by the ADEQ, one for exceeding the arsenic drinking water standard. In the words of a *Gardenroots* participant: "The people in Humboldt served by Humboldt Water System are deeply indebted to Mrs. Ramirez-Andreotta's study which served to reveal a serious problem with the municipal water." Additionally, arsenic concentrations in water exceeded the drinking water standard for several participants who rely solely on their private wells for potable water. UA personnel worked closely with those households to provide information regarding water treatment technologies that could be implemented to reduce their arsenic concentrations. Now, the community is reporting that they are regularly testing their private wells, and are encouraging ADEQ to ensure that water entering their home is at or below the arsenic drinking water standard.

Furthermore, *Gardenroots* built trust between the UA scientists and the Dewey-Humboldt, Arizona community. This trust has set the groundwork for a long-term community-academic partnership. Due to the efforts discussed above, three additional research projects have been initiated to address pressing remediation and characterization challenges posed by the Iron King site. For example, the Metals Exposure Study in Homes was designed to determine the levels of metal exposure in children ages 1-11 years. Two former *Gardenroots* participants have been hired as UA employees to be part of the local field team. This is evidence that the *Gardenroots* community-academic partnership has enhanced social capital and community capacity and has even had a small economic impact in the community.

Discussion

Several limitations were observed throughout the project and these are also presented in table 1. First, setting and maintaining the expectations was a challenging. For example, *Gardenroots* could provide environmental monitoring and potential soil, water and vegetable exposure data, but could not provide specific data related to health outcomes. It was important to restate the goals and what type of data could truly be expected from the project. Second, due to the nature of the sample analyses and formal laboratory procedures, the participants did not get to prepare and analyze their own samples. In response, participants were invited to a laboratory tour called "The Science Behind *Gardenroots*" at the UA to learn the methodologies. Unfortunately, the attendance was low, and this was most likely due to the travel distance (~200 miles) and large time commitment. Lastly, even though *Gardenroots* informed the USEPA and ADEQ on all activities, it was challenging to maintain bidirectional communication between the *Gardenroots* project leader and all government agencies working at the site. At one point, EPA did not agree with the communication methodology, was uncomfortable with a few community member's responses and activism (Ramirez-Andreotta et al., forthcoming).

Reflecting on the process

Gardenroots satisfied the concepts of a co-created citizen project (co-created PPSR) based upon the level of participation throughout the scientific research process (Table 1), as compared to a contributory project (where participants solely collect samples) or a collaborative project (were participants may be involved in five or more additional steps) (12). In addition, *Gardenroots* was a CBPR project that, as originally outline by Israel et al., 1998, recognized the community as an unit of identity, facilitated collaborative, equitable involvement of all partners in most phases of the research, integrated knowledge and intervention for mutual benefit of all partners, promoted a co-learning and empowering process, and disseminated findings and knowledge gained to all partners. There are more components involved in CBPR, but not all projects require or are functionally set up to involve each and every component. It is important to be flexible and adapt to what is actually feasible, while successfully meeting and maintaining the expectations of the community-academic partnership.

In addition to describing risk, practitioners must also put the risk into perspective and in terms of consumption behavior. Converting the raw risk data into a personalized, more relatable format, specifically the quantity of vegetables they could consume at various target risks, and comparing this exposure route to water and soil ingestion was instrumental in translating the *Gardenroots* results. It is recommended that participants be given all of their personal data to review so that they can then decide for themselves which risk level is comfortable for them. This act can also facilitate inquiry and knowledge synthesis where participants compare and combine the results with their existing knowledge, furthering their inquiry-based learning.

Public participation methods have been used for a few exposure assessment and health studies, but not in conjunction with risk communication at a Superfund site. This case study demonstrates that risk communication efforts can be effective when the affected community is involved in the research project and in determining the content of the risk analysis. In addition, evaluating program outcomes at the individual, programmatic, and community levels is a useful and creative way to capture the successes of citizen science and community-academic partnerships.

In summary, the project design clearly justifies public participation in scientific research projects, hopefully may influence national policy regarding environmental science education practices for the general public, and definitely redefines who may generate environmental monitoring data in site assessments.

Acknowledgments

The authors would like to give a special thanks to all the *Gardenroots* participants for their participation and assistance in the project and for reviewing this manuscript. Additionally, the authors would like to thank the town of Dewey-Humboldt, Arizona, Jeff Franklin, Dewey-Humboldt Town Librarian, Jeff Schalau, UA Yavapai Cooperative Extension Director, Mike Kopplin, UA Superfund Research Program's Hazard Identification Core, and Dr. Atasi Ray-Maitra, UA Water Quality Laboratory. Lastly, thank you to Dr. Phil Brown for his comments on this manuscript.

This research was funded by the US EPA Office of Research and Development and NIEHS' Superfund Research Program (Grant P42 ES04940). The first author gratefully acknowledges financial support by the NASA Space Grant Program, UA TRIF Water Sustainability Program, and the Alfred P. Sloan Foundation that funds the National Action Council for Minorities in Engineering Scholarship program.

Supplemental Material

Supplemental Material Table 1. Demographics of *Gardenroots* participants (N=18)

Demographics	Percentage
Gender	
Male	37
Female	63
Age (years)	
18 – 28	5.0
29 – 39	5.0
40 – 49	11
50 – 59	37
60 – 69	32
70 – 79	5.0
80+	0
Last academic Experience	
High School	22
Community College, Associates Degree	33
University/College, Bachelor's Degree	17
University/College, Masters/PhD	11
Trade/Technical School/Training Program	11
Years living in the area	
0 – 2 years	21
3 – 5 years	26
6 – 8 years	16
8+ years	37

Note: Percentages adding to less than 100% signifies missing data.

Location	Target Risk 1/1,000,000	Target Risk 1/100,000	Target Risk 1/10,000	USDA Recommended Amount (cups/week)
Onion				
Your Garden	3/4	7	70	4 cups/week total of "Other Vegetables"
Lettuce				
Your Garden	1/2	5	50	3 cups/week total of "Raw Leafy Dark Green Vegetables"
Tomato				
Your Garden	1-1/2	15	150	5 cups/week of "red and orange vegetables"

This is just an example; no actual community member results are shown.

Supplemental Figure 1. Amount you can eat from your garden based on a varying cancer target risk. An example of the risk communication and graphical layout selected to inform and properly answer the research question posed by the community: "How much can I eat from my garden?"

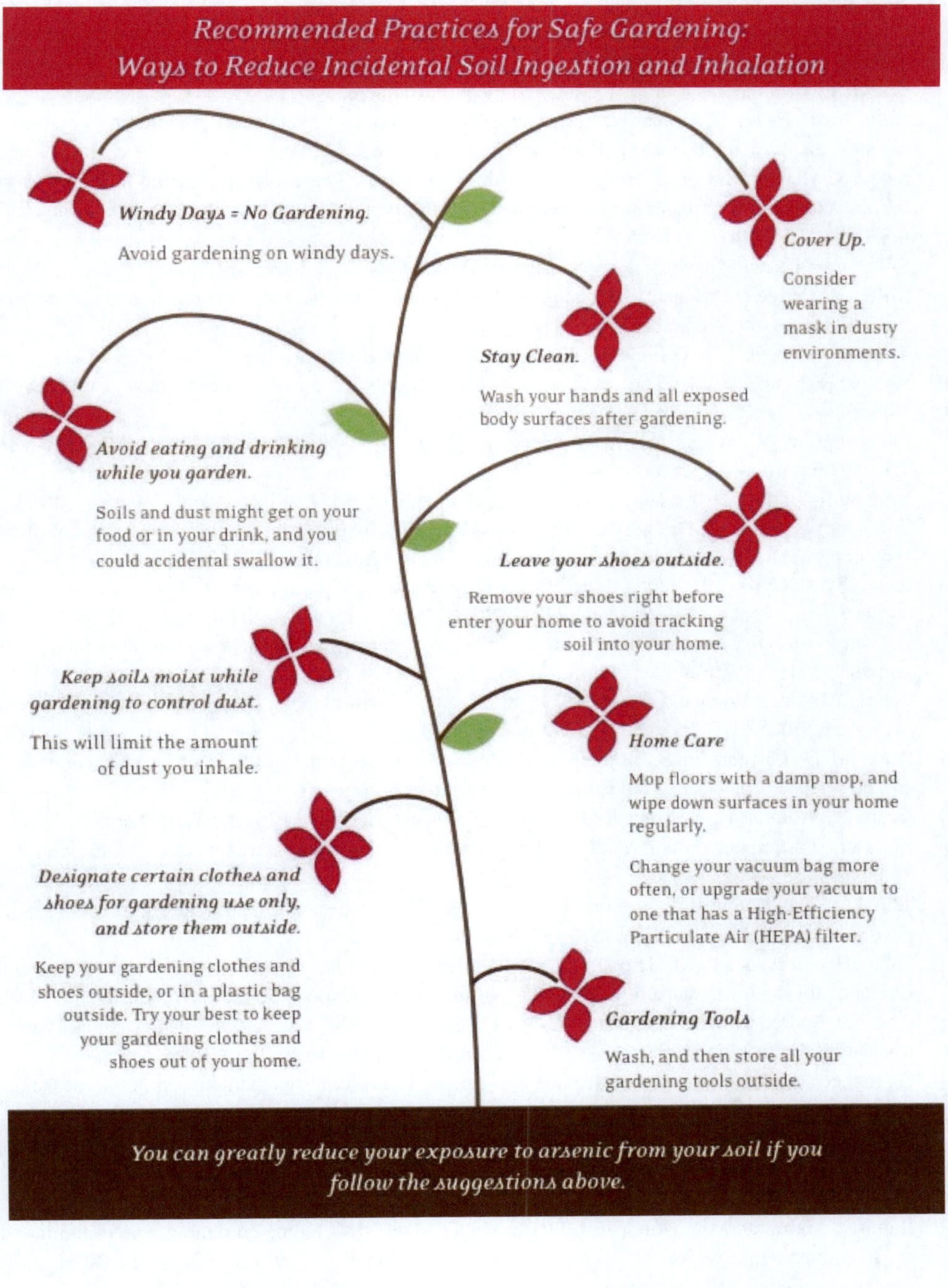

Supplemental Figure 2. An example of one of the three waterproof handouts that were made to disseminate the recommended behavioral modifications necessary to reduce arsenic exposure.

References

[1] Brown P, Mikkelsen EJ. No safe place. Toxic waste, leukemia, and community action. Berkeley, CA: University California Press, 1990.

[2] National Research Council. Alternatives for managing the nation's complex contaminated groundwater sites. Washington, DC: National Academy Press, 2012.

[3] Chess C, Purchell K. Public participation and the environment. Do we know what works? Environ Sci Technol 1999;30(16):2685-92.

[4] Cox R. Environmental communication and the public sphere. Thosand Oaks, CA: Sage, 2013.

[5] Galvez MP, Peters R, Graber N, Forman J. Effective risk communication in children's environmental health. Lessons learned from 9/11. Pediatr Clin North Am 2007;54:33-46.

[6] Senier L, Hudson B, Fort S, Hoover E, Tillson R, Brown P. The Brown Superfund Research Program. A multistakeholder partnership addresses real-world problems in contaminated communities. Environ Sci Technol 2008;42(13):4655-62.

[7] Silbertown J. A new dawn for citizen science. Trends Ecol Evol 2009;24(9):467-71.

[8] Miller-Rushing A, Primack R, Bonney R. The history of public participation in ecological research. Front Ecol Environ 2012;10(6)285-90.

[9] Thoits PA, Hewitt LN. Volunteer work and well-being. J Health Soc Behav 2001;42:115–31.

[10] Wilson J, Musick M. The effects of volunteering on the volunteer. Law Contemp Probl 1999;62(4):141–68.

[11] Flemming W. Volunteer watershed health monitoring by local stakeholders. New MexicoWatershed Watch. J Environ Educ 2003;35(1):27–32.

[12] Bonney R, Ballard H, Jordan R, McCallie E, Phillips T, Shirk J, Wilderman CC. Public Participation in Scientific Research: Defining the Field and Assessing Its Potential for Informal Science Education. Washington, DC: Center Advancement Informal Science Education (CAISE), 2009.

[13] Israel BA, Schulz AJ, Parker EA, Becker AB. Review of community-based research. Assessing partnership approaches to improve public health. Annu Rev Public Health 1998;19:173–202.

[14] Brown P. Popular epidemiology and toxic waste contamination. Lay and professional ways of knowing. J Health Soc Behav 1992;33(3):267-81.

[15] Corburn J. Street science. Community knowledge and environmental health justice. CAmbridge, MA: MIT Press, 2005.

[16] Brossard D, Lewenstein B, Bonney R. Scientific knowledge and attitude change. The impact of a citizen science project. Int J Sci Educ 2005;27(9):1099–121.

[17] Evans C, Abrams E, Reitsma R, Roux K, Salmonsen L, Marra PP. The Neighborhood Nestwatch Program. Participant outcomes of a citizen science ecological research project. Conservation Biol 2005;19(3):589-94.

[18] Trumbull DJ, Bonney R, Bascom D, Cabral A. Thinking scientifically during participation in a citizen-science project. Sci Educ 2000;84:265–75.

[19] Falk JH, Storksdieck M, Dierking LD. Investigating public science interest and understanding. Evidence for the importance of free-choice learning. Public Underst Sci 2007;16:455-69.

[20] Ramirez-Andreotta MD, Brusseau ML, Artiola JF, Maier RM, Gandolfi AJ. Environmental research translation. Enhancing interactions with communities at contaminated sites, forthcoming.

[21] Gallagher DR. Advocates for environmental justice. The role of the champion in public participation. Local Environ 2009;14(10):905-16.

[22] Green L, Fullilove M, Evans D, Shepard P. "Hey, Mom, thanks!" Use of focus groups in the development of place-specific materials for a community environmental action campaign. Environ Health Perspect 2002;110(2):265–9.

[23] Ramirez-Andreotta MD, Brusseau ML, Beamer P, Maier RM. Home gardening near a mining site in an arsenic-endemic region of Arizona. Assessing arsenic exposure and risk via ingestion of home garden vegetables, soils and potable water. Sci Total Environ 2013;454-455:373–82.

[24] Jordan RC, Ballard HL, Phillips TB. Key issues and new approaches for evaluating citizen-science learning outcomes. Front Ecol Environ 2012;10(6):307-9.

[25] Brown P, Brody JG, Morello-Forsch R, Tovar J, Zota AR, Rudel RA. Measuring the success of community science. The Northern California Household Exposure Study. Environ Health Perspect 2012;120(3):326-31.

[26] Baron S, Sinclair R, Payne-Sturges D, Phelps J, Zenick H, Collman GW, et al. Partnerships for environmental and occupational justice. Contributions to research, capacity and public health. Am J Public Health 2009;99(Suppl 3):S517–25.

[27] Adams C, Brown P, Morello-Frosch R, Brody JG, Rudel R, Zota A, et al. Disentangling the exposure experience. The roles of community context and report-back of environmental exposure data. J Health Soc Behav 2011;52(2):180–96.

[28] Ramirez-Andreotta MD, Brusseau ML, Artiola JF, Maier RM. A greenhouse and field-based study to determine the accumulation of arsenic in common homegrown vegetables. Sci Total Environ 2013;433:299-306.

[29] Brody JG, Morello-Frosch R, Brown P, Rudel RA, Altman RG, Frye M, et al. Improving disclosure and consent: "is it safe?": new ethics for reporting personal exposures to environmental chemicals. Am J Public Health 2007;97(9):1547-54.

In: Public Health
Editors: Rosemary M. Caron and Joav Merrick

ISBN: 978-1-63321-569-6

Chapter 16

Bridging organizations in promoting health

Paivi Abernethy*
Department of Environment and Resource Studies, University of Waterloo, Waterloo, Canada

Promoting health has remained strongly in the domain of the health sector, despite the ambitious rhetoric of international agreements. Complex environmental health issues, for instance, are not solvable without active collaboration of the public, private, not-for-profit, and academic sectors together with the communities in which they function. This paper explored the United Nations Educational, Scientific and Cultural Organization (UNESCO) mandated biosphere reserves as bridging organizations outside of the health sector that have begun to bring together diverse stakeholders to address public health and environmental issues as an integrated part of sustainability. A qualitative study of Canadian and British biosphere reserves revealed cross-sectoral health promoting projects ranging from individual health behavior change to those embracing wider social determinants of health. Drivers for and barriers to the integration work were analyzed. Results indicate that organizations with primary focus other than health have a potential to play a meaningful role in providing a neutral, apolitical, platform that helps bringing diverse community stakeholders to the table to promote health.

Introduction

Promoting health has remained strongly in the domain of the health sector, despite the ambitious rhetoric of international agreements such as 'Bangkok Charter for Health Promotion' (1) and 'Health in All Policies' (2) that declared health as a responsibility of all sectors. Environmental health is an area where health outcomes cannot be the sole responsibility of the health sector. Complex environmental issues are not solvable without

* Corresponding author: Paivi Abernethy, PhD Candidate, MSc, MRes, Environment and Resources Studies, University of Waterloo, 200 University Avenue West, Waterloo, ON N2L 3G1, Canada. E-mail: pkaberne@uwaterloo.ca.

active collaboration of the public, private, not-for-profit, and academic sectors together with the communities in which they function. Furthermore, environmental pollution and other social determinants of health, such as food security and sustainable livelihoods, are interests shared by diverse health and environmental stakeholders, as well as communities in general.

In current compartmentalized societies, however, someone needs to take the initiative to cross the disciplinary or interest-specific boundaries. Often neither health professionals nor environmental authorities see themselves as having the mandate or capacity to take the lead in addressing environmental health issues. Non-governmental organizations, however, have a greater flexibility in directing their activities. Social movements and organizations addressing specific social determinants of health are known to facilitate cross-sectoral collaborations, such as the 'Vibrant Communities' initiatives focusing on poverty reduction (3). A Dutch study (4), explored health brokers as specific agents facilitating cross-sectoral health promotion. There has been little study of organizations whose cross-sectoral mandates are only implicitly health-related, yet sufficient as a basis for bringing together diverse stakeholders to promote health. This paper explores the potential of UNESCO mandated biosphere reserves (BRs) as bridging organizations bringing together communities for health and sustainable development

A BR is a specific region, recognized by UNESCO, guided by an organization of the same name that attempts to help people find ways to build sustainable livelihoods while maintaining the health of the ecosystem that supports their existence within the area (5). Currently, there are 621 BRs in 117 countries (6). The structure, organization and governance of BRs have been adapted to meet the local conditions and needs and therefore vary significantly from one another (7). Because of their mandate, BRs are often viewed as 'learning laboratories' for sustainable development (8-9). The purpose of BRs is to demonstrate the integration of conservation and sustainable development.

In this study, BRs were analyzed as examples of organizations outside of the health sector that have begun to bring together diverse stakeholders to address public health and environmental issues as an integrated part of sustainability. Because of the local adaptations of the mandate, only some BRs have included health promotion explicitly in their operations. This study explored how and why some BRs have explicitly integrated health into their activities, whilst others have not. Furthermore, it investigated the types of health related programming as well as drivers for and barriers to implementing health focus.

'Bridging organizations' is a new concept to health promotion and public health but is used in, for example, international development (10) and environmental governance (11-13) literatures. The term refers to local groups or associations that facilitate horizontal linkages between sectors as well as foster vertical connections across administrative layers, which allow local influence on higher level decision-making and policy development (10). The Millennium Ecosystem Assessment (14) defined their purpose as to facilitate collaboration among actors by providing "arenas for multisector and/or multilevel collaboration for conceiving visions, trust-building, collaboration, learning, value formation, conflict resolution, and other institutional innovations". Bridging organizations are often seen critical for community capacity-building (14) and for adaptive co-management of natural resources (15), because they provide both services and facilitate collaboration between non-governmental organizations, government agencies, research organizations, and other stakeholders.

The Millennium Ecosystem Assessment as well as adaptive environmental governance literature, in general, have identified BRs as bridging organizations (11-12,14). The role of BRs as bridging organizations is to create a safe meeting forum to facilitate cross-sectoral collaboration (13,17-18). Many BRs appear also to be functioning as bridging organizations in practice. Forty-six of 146 surveyed BR managers said their organizations were "effectively achieving developmental goals" by engaging local stakeholders, academics, politicians and government administrators in sustainable development and conservation promotion (18). This study by Schultz et al. emphasized the great potential role of BRs as bridging organization in linking ecosystem services and human well-being, which is a complex, long-term, experiment requiring continuous innovation and learning.

The factors influencing health and well-being extend from biophysical to socioeconomic elements, thus finding meaningful, sustainable solutions to the complex public health challenges requires complex solutions. Already in 1973, Rittel and Webber (19) labeled these complicated, messy challenges as 'wicked problems' and the discussion has been on-going. By their nature, environmental health issues fall under this category (20-22). They involve a great range of stakeholders, who perceive the problem and its solutions in various ways. Wicked problems can be managed, if not solved (21), but that requires natural scientific as well as social scientific understanding and solution alternatives. Because wicked problems often are created by pigeonholed problem solving attempts, tackling them demands opening up for new ways of thinking (22). This paper explores one unconventional, alternative approach to facilitating cross-sectoral collaboration to promote public health that addresses limitations of the current system.

Our project

The research project focused on cross-sectoral bridging of health and sustainable development. This particular component of the study centered on asking: How can non-governmental organizations function as bridging agents facilitating cross-sectoral collaboration between the health and environmental sectors? The data were collected by document analyses, semi-structured interviews and, overt participant observation. The analysis was made by analytic induction (23), using sensitizing concepts based on health promotion theories to frame the investigation with the desired focus (see table 1) (23). The research aimed to find answers to the following four questions: 1) What type of health promotion related activities and programs take place in the BRs? 2) To what extent have the BRs been able to function as bridging agents facilitating cross-sectoral collaboration between health and sustainability sectors? 3) What type of barriers to and drivers for integrating health into their programming can be identified? This research followed the normal procedures for health research concerning human participants with full ethics clearance by the Office of Research Ethics at the University of Waterloo (ORE #18477).

Explicitly health-related projects were investigated in all Canadian (n=16) and British (n=3) BRs that follow the guidelines specified by the Madrid Action Plan (24). The Canadian analysis was based on a project database created by Helene Godmaire of the Canadian BR Association (CBRA), semi-structured interviews, and participant observation at two Annual General Meetings of CBRA, in 2011 and 2012, respectively. The British analysis was based on document analysis, semi-structured interviews, and one week of participant observation in the two established BRs.

Table 1. Examples of how *health* and *well-being* were addressed in Madrid Action Plan (24)

The potential role of BRs in addressing emerging challenges caused by climate change, biodiversity loss, and rapid urbanization (p.4):
• "From these challenges, several opportunities for change arise, through increased awareness at all levels of the need to maintain and secure access to ecosystem services for human **well-being**, including **health**, security and justice/equity." • "Develop mechanisms to encourage the sustainable development of BRs carried out in partnership with all sectors of society (i.e. public and private institutions, [non-governmental organizations], stakeholder communities, decision- makers, scientists, local and indigenous communities, land owners and users of natural resources, research and education centres, media) to ensure the **well-being** of people and their environment;…" [emphasis added]
The Madrid Action Plan's overall goals are to (p.5):
• "anchor the research, training, capacity building and demonstration agendas of [Man and the Biosphere-project] at the interface between the interlinked issues of conservation and sustainable use of biodiversity, mitigation and adaptation to climate change, and socio-economic and cultural **well-being** of human communities" • "enable the active use of places included in the [World Network of Biosphere Reserves] as learning sites for sustainable development, i.e. demonstrating approaches to enhance co-operation amongst epistemic (academic), political, practitioner and stakeholder communities to address and solve context specific problems to improve environmental, economic and social conditions for human and ecosystem **well-being**" [emphasis added]

North Devon, Dyfi, Frontenac Arch, and Georgian Bay BRs were selected for detailed case studies to identify all activities that can be considered health promotion, and to understand the collaborative relationships, drivers for, and barriers to the integration of health into programming. The selection was based on three criteria: two case studies per country; two organizations that had programming with an explicit health focus and two that did not focus on health; and comparability of their geographic profiles.

Semi-structured interviews (n=29) were conducted at all four locations between November 2012 and May 2013. The interviewees were all experts in the field, staff, partners or Board members of the BRs, and therefore the qualitative in-depth interviews followed an inter-active style (23). The interview guide covered four specific areas: health-related projects, barriers to and drivers for health integration, available local knowledge, and cross-sectoral bridging capacity. The order and format of the questions varied depending on the flow of the discussion and the professional role of the interviewee. Interviews were conducted until saturation was observed and the same topics kept reappearing in responses.

Data analysis

All the interviews were recorded and transcribed by the author. The coding was created based on sensitizing concepts and additional codes were created when unanticipated health promotion related topics appeared. Participants were provided with a summary of all findings and specifics related to their own interviews for review and validation. Triangulation of the results was further strengthened by engaging other health promotion professionals to assess the analysis and appropriateness of coding. Because of the rural and small community context, all the results have been pooled to one single general story of BRs as bridging organizations for health and sustainable development to protect the confidentiality and relative anonymity of the participants

Findings

The results come successively from the pilot project and the case studies. The pilot component of the project explored the status of health in the universal UNESCO mandate and in the activities of BRs. Attitudes towards health-related activities among BR practitioners were also explored. The pilot results provided justification to the four in-depth case studies.

Document analysis and participant observation assessing health focus in the UNESCO mandate, in general, and in Canadian and British BRs in particular The 3rd World Congress of BRs, held in February 2008, produced the 'Madrid Action Plan' for the BRs. It can be considered as the overall strategic mandate for BRs for 2008-2013. Building on the Seville Strategy of 1995 that shifted the focus from conservation to sustainable development, the Madrid Action Plan aimed "to raise BRs to be the principal internationally-designated areas dedicated to sustainable development in the 21st century."(24). In the document, the words health and well-being show up once and ten times, respectively (see table 1).

Well-being is also included in both vision and mission statements for the 'World Network of BRs', which aim:

- To foster "harmonious integration of people and nature for sustainable development through participatory dialogue, knowledge sharing, poverty reduction and human well-being improvements, respect for cultural values and society's ability to cope with change, thus contributing to the [Millennium Development Goals]"; and
- "To ensure environmental, economic, social (including cultural and spiritual) sustainability through: development and coordination of a worldwide network of places acting as demonstration areas and learning sites with the aim of maintaining and developing ecological and cultural diversity, and securing ecosystem services for human well-being".

Many BRs mention health on their website, promoting healthy economy, healthy environment, healthy society, and healthy culture (e.g. Bras d'Or Lake BR and Georgian Bay BR). However, only two out of the sixteen BRs in Canada and one out of the original two (now three) in the UK explicitly addressed human health in their activities, when the research project was embarked in 2011. When asked about their interest in integrating health in biosphere activities, organisations that did not explicitly focus on health expressed a unanimous desire to learn more about the opportunities to collaborate with the public health sector. Only one of the studied BRs, Clayoquot Sound BR, has adopted healthy communities as one of its three core priorities and also extensively focuses on health in its activities. The BR is located on Nuu-chah-nulths First Nations' traditional lands, who represent fifty per cent of the current all-year population in the area. Originally the Western term sustainable development was replaced by healthy communities, but nowadays the terms appear interchangeably in the Clayoquot public documents. Clayoquot Sound BR is also the only one of all the Canadian and British BRs studied that explicitly defines health on its website:

> "Health encompasses everything from walking trails and clean water to access to recreational opportunities, adequate housing and stable employment. The [Clayoquot Biosphere Trust] is committed to supporting projects that support health, in its broadest sense." (clayoquotbiosphere.org; emphasis added)

These findings were deemed sufficient to advance to the four case studies, which is the main focus of this paper.

Further document analysis, semi-structured interviews, and participant observation, focusing on the four cases studies

Almost all activities in the Canadian and British BRs depend on project specific grants from private foundations or governments. Moreover, most of the activities rely on community volunteers and are supported by in kind contributions from partnering organizations. The actual operational funding of the BRs is relatively small and reflected in the number of paid staff, which ranges from two part-time individuals to five full-time employees in the BRs in question. Only one of the four organizations has a full-time paid manager. One BR has two paid part-time managers sharing the duty, and two BRs have volunteer-based management. The staffing and funding structures vary from region to region. In 2012, federal government prematurely terminated five-year operational funding support for the Canadian BRs, as part of the broader financial cuts to the environmental sector. One of the three BRs in the UK operates autonomously under the Regional Council; the other two are essentially grassroots organizations, despite their UNESCO status. All four case study organizations perceive themselves as partnerships or networks and see the role of their staff to function as networking facilitators, who bring together partners to work on shared issues. The following table (see table 2) provides an overview of the types of health promotion related activities that have taken place within the four BRs, since adaptation to the Seville Strategy. Mapping all the projects and involved partners of the BRs was beyond the scope of this project, but table 2 helps illustrate the range of identified health-related activities as well as the scope of bridging potential that this type of organizations may hold. The sensitizing concepts were based on generally accepted health promotion categories and concepts (25-26). They acknowledge health promotion efforts needed at multiple levels of the society, from facilitating the individual behavior change to systems-wide policy change, as well as the impact of social determinants of health. Some examples could fit under multiple categories but they are included only once to illustrate the diversity. BRs aim to remain politically neutral and therefore the organizations do not engage in advocacy and direct policy development activities.

Table 2. Health promotion projects in BRs since the adaptation to the Seville Strategy

Health promotion category	Examples of projects related to public health	Types of partners engaged
PROMOTING HEALTHY BEHAVIOUR CHANGE		
A) Focus on individual behaviour change		
Physical activity	"Walking for Health": local walking groups that provide walks specifically tailored to support good health through exercise and social interaction; e.g., tinyurl.com/WalkingGroups [accessed 2014 Jan 15]	Public health (NHS*), local governments, ENGOs*, other NGOs*, community volunteers
Nutrition (physical activity)	"Local Flavours": a program promoting local food production and healthy, nutritious eating, combined with local art, and connecting food and nutrition with physical activity; includes over 100 local food producers, retailers, and food services; e.g., tinyurl.com/LocalFlavours & tinyurl.com/ActiveBody [accessed 2014 Jan 15]	Public health unit (nutritionist), local governments, private the private sector, ENGOs*, community volunteers
Nutrition	Free, food-related, community workshops in collaboration with local volunteers: growing own fresh food, identifying edible wild plants, raising chicken & keeping bees; e.g., tinyurl.com/BR-ActionGroup & tinyurl.com/GrowOwnFood [accessed 2014 Jan 15]	Public health unit (community health promoter); HNGO* (intellectual disabilities); other NGOs*, community volunteers
Environmental health	"Life on the Bay": guidance for healthy & sustainable septic tank management, handling of domestic toxic chemicals, drinking water & waste treatment, etc.; e.g., tinyurl.com/EnvGuide [accessed 2014 Jan 15]	Federal & provincial governments (Parks Canada, Environment Canada, Ontario MNR*), the private sector, and ENGOs*
Mental health (physical activity)	"Tirwedd Dyfi": promoting well-being gained by understanding the linkages between the sense of place, language, culture, landscape and being outdoors; focus on lifestyles; "trying to get people to appreciate the importance of the outdoors in Welsh language culture, in other words tempt them to go out and to see the outside and landscape as being part of their innate culture…" (interview participant); e.g. tinyurl.com/HealthyCulture & tinyurl.com/CulturePaths [accessed 2014 Jan 15]	National & regional governments (National Park Authority & CCW*), schools, ENGOs* & other NGOs*, community volunteers
B) Focus on community level behaviour change		
Food security	Cookbook supporting local foods: emphasizing what people eat and how its produced leaves lasting traces in the local landscape and culture,	University of the Third Age, NGOs*, the private sector

Table 2. (Continued)

Health promotion category	Examples of projects related to public health	Types of partners engaged
	connecting food with the living and working countryside; e.g., tinyurl.com/CookLocal [accessed 2014 Jan 15]	
Food security	Interactive collaborative school program to promote local food, engaging children to analyse the local food system and engage the community in their research; e.g., tinyurl.com/Food-Kids [accessed 2014 Jan 15]	Schools, university, government, ENGOs*, other NGOs*, local food producers & the private sector
Active transportation (nutrition/ food security)	Interactive trails maps with health messaging & sustainable development focus; e.g. bringing together over 30 regional trail organizations; e.g., tinyurl.com/TrailNetwork & tinyurl.com/ActiveWithNature [accessed 2014 Jan 15]	Public health, federal & provincial governments (Parks Canada; Ontario Parks, MTCS*, MOE*, & MNR*), municipal governments, ENGOs*, other NGOs*, the private sector, community volunteers
Active transportation	Easy access trail mapping project to promote active transportation and outdoors experiences to mobility challenged individuals; e.g. tinyurl.com/EasyTrails [accessed 2014 Jan 15]	ENGOs*, HNGO* (physical disabilities), local governments, community volunteers
Environmental Health	"Catchment Sensitive Farming": a partnership to reduce diffuse pollution from agriculture& grant management; e.g. tinyurl.com/HealthyFarming & tinyurl.com/ FarmingGrants [accessed 2014 Jan 15]	ENGOs*, national government (Environment Agency), local farmers
PROMOTING SYSTEMS LEVEL CHANGE		
Food security (poverty reduction)	Collaborating to expand the existing community gardens, providing workshops (see above example A3), arranging "Food Festivals" and a "Food Forum" to create awareness and to develop a sustainable food system as part of poverty reduction efforts & sustainable community development [in rural communities efforts are often intertwined]; e.g., tinyurl.com/LocalFoodMap & tinyurl.com/ LocalFoodsystem & tinyurl.com/ HealthyUrbanForest [accessed 2014 Jan 15]	Public health (community health promoter), local hospital, HNGO* (intellectual disabilities); other NGOs*, municipal government, community volunteers
Healthy & sustainable	Initiating and organizing a "Regional Sustainability Initiative", a "Community Survey" and "Integrated Community Sustainability	Public health (MOH*), health professionals (family physicians),

Health promotion category	Examples of projects related to public health	Types of partners engaged
community development	Plans", inviting a broad range of community stakeholders to the table; e.g., tinyurl.com/AskingCommunity & tinyurl.com/BRdrivenICSP & tinyurl.com/ CrossSectoralCollaboration [accessed 2014 Jan 15]	local municipalities, public library, ENGOs*, HNGO* (developmental disabilities), other NGOs*, school boards, the private sector
Environmental health (Poverty reduction)	"Sustainable Energy Action Plan and Sustainable Energy Partnership": including public, private and voluntary sector interests and education/training providers; coordinating strategic planning and action towards zero carbon energy use goal (includes tackling fuel poverty); e.g., tinyurl.com/SustEnergyPlan & tinyurl.com/ CommPartnerships [accessed 2014 Jan 15]	A broad range of the public & private sector stakeholders, NGOs, *schools, public housing, etc.
Environmental health	"State of the Bay": ecosystem health report card; presents information about key ecosystem health indicators along the Bay. Key indicators were selected in the areas of water quality, wetlands, fisheries, and landscape; summarizes existing scientific reports from the local perspective; e.g. preview.tinyurl.com/EnvAssessment [accessed 2014 Jan 15]	5 other local ENGOs*; federal & provincial governments (funding)

[*NGO: Non-Governmental Organization; ENGO: Environmental NGO; HNGO; Health-related NGO; MOH: Medical Officer of Health; CCW: Countryside Council for Wales, currently known as Natural Resources Wales; NHS: UK National Health Services; MNR: Ontario Ministry of Natural Resources; MOE: Ontario Ministry of Environment; MTCS: Ontario Ministry of Tourism, Culture and Sports].

To assess the future potential of the BRs as bridging organizations bringing together health and sustainability the key drivers for and barriers to such integration processes were explored. Some of the main topics identified can be found in table 3 with examples of the responses categorized under respective themes.

Table 3. Participant comments on barriers to and drivers for integrating health and sustainable development

Drivers for & barriers to integrating health	Identified themes and examples of verbatim quotes from interview responses
Health being explicit vs. implicit in mandate/ activities	• **Not explicit:** "It's may be in the BR's vision statement (…) – but it's not explicit in the strategic level of what the BR is doing, that it should be promoting health. I think there is a natural kind of overlap, but the priorities that have been set don't spell it out…"

Table 3. (Continued)

Drivers for & barriers to integrating health	Identified themes and examples of verbatim quotes from interview responses
	• **Disadvantage of health not being explicit:** "If we're not being pulled in a health direction, it might not be spelled out as that, it might not be identified as that, or it might not happen." • **Value of making health explicit:** "If you think that public health is part of sustainability, these are some of the areas that would be particularly relevant and these could maybe some of the techniques that could be used." • **Supportive vs. active role:** "happy to encourage [health promotion]. (…) But I don't see my role, at the moment, to initiate that sort of project."
Knowledge & awareness	• **Unawareness within the health sector:** "Going to health meetings where there is absolutely no interest at all – they talk about healthy foods and healthy eating – but there is no interest at all to what food is produced [here] – or no knowledge. There is no attempt at choosing local produce." • **Unawareness within the BR:** "It's the individuals who sort of shape the organization. Take a look at our Board, it's the same thing. If [the health researcher interviewing] were to join our Board then you would introduce new ideas and new concepts and help us explore new ideas. If it isn't there, it is not part of the organisation background – in terms of the people that are involved." • **Understanding within the BR:** "From the data point of view, if you look at the statistics of the BR, you can see that there is a lot of deprivation and disease. That data has been collected nationally, so we can compare ourselves as a region with the rest of the county or country. We can even interpolate between these data points, since it's all based on national health statistics and census data. So we can see that in the BR region there are some real critical health and economy issues for a lot of people. Superimposing another data set that explored the sense of pride people in their area, their likely health status according the stats, their income, all these three things overlap geographically and correlate really well. In other words a person will no interest in their area, is likely to be have low income, and highly likely to suffer an illness."
Perception	• **Health as a driver for sustainability:** "If we look at human wellbeing as the driver of sustainable development and the driver of individual's position within sustainable development, then you could say that their own personal health and economic and social wellbeing is a key factor in how a community wellbeing is built up. (…) Theoretically and strategically it's all there, but operationally it gets a bit challenging" • **Lack of general awareness:** "I think [the interconnectedness between health and sustainable development] is explicit but getting the awareness – how would it come? • **Polarized perspectives:** "You get two camps – this is mostly the scientific measurable stuff and we do all that, and then we have a group of people who are all about process and the emotional wellbeing (…), the personal health. Obviously health is both."

Drivers for & barriers to integrating health	Identified themes and examples of verbatim quotes from interview responses
Community champions and networking	• **Among the professionals/ practitioners:** "[The Medical Officer of Health] down here has really kind of knitted together a health unit enterprise and brought diverse groups into large and more cohesive units. And her focus is to work with the community." • **In the community:** "People in this area don't like to push themselves. They're naturally shy and whenever you have a public meeting, you always find that the hall will fill up from the back to the front. Nobody wants to sit in the front row and this is something we have to recognise (…) You have to identify those individuals in the community who are naturally more assertive to speak up on their behalf." • **Cross-sectoral bridging:** "Then again [the public health staff] will decide 'what resources do we have in our area, if they can help us [reach our operational goals]. 'Oh the BR s here – what can we do to encourage people to use their trails?' (…) we can do [health promotion] together. (…) So that's how it would happen from our end. Then from their end, they might say 'we're really interested in this' and then [the 'champion' from the BR] would speak to me and I would say 'sounds like a fit with what we're doing. I'll give you [Z]'s name' – and he knows [Z] cause she's one of the public health nurses – 'why don't the two of you talk together if we can actually make that happen'. So it would happen both ways."
Funding/ time	• **Operational funding challenge:** "I can go to a [granting body] and (…) probably get somebody to do healthy communities. Say if you have a contingency of three or four staff and you want to keep them going. As a manager, you are managing those folks but you are also trying to ensure that there is continuity – so that grant follows grant follows grant, so you can keep them on-board. (…) Capacity issue is a pretty significant issue. Because you're still also trying to do all that outreach. We should be able to take the organisation to another level to be able to take on-board a healthy communities coordinator. [That requires] adding some management time, but where does that money come from."

Discussion

The in-depth interviews, analysis of public documents, and participant observations, summarized above, indicate that, albeit not explicit, the universal UNESCO mandate appears to support efforts promoting health and well-being. Moreover, a great range of projects undertaken by BR organizations fall under the umbrella of health promotion (see table 2). The projects have involved both health-related activities that focus more narrowly on individual health behavior change, such as physical activity, and those that address key social determinants of health, including poverty and food security.

All the participants in the case studies saw health and sustainable development as inherently interlinked topics, although most of the interviewees felt that the connection was intuitive rather than explainable. Individual interpretations of this interwovenness were strongly influenced by professional backgrounds, but the ubiquitous perception of interconnectedness creates a promising platform potential for increased practical integration of health and sustainability.

Three out of the four case organizations have bridged health and sustainable development by engaging health stakeholders. The fourth BR has indirect engagement through its core partner organizations, which have active collaboration with the health sector. The greatest range of health promotional activities could be identified when the BR had direct collaboration with the administrative top-level of health organizations. Although it was not always explicitly expressed, all case-study BRs have health promotion programs related to both individual health behavior change and systems change addressing wider social determinants of health (see table 2).

All participating organizations noted that the interest of local individuals is the main determining factor for addressing health-related issues. Despite the differences in organizational structures (three organizations being strictly non-governmental and one functioning as an autonomous entity within the regional council), all four biospheres have interpreted their responsibility under the UNESCO mandate as building, in an inclusive manner from bottom-up, on local assets and needs. This deliberative approach, which is supported in much of the community-based health promotion literature (27-28), fosters the local issue ownership vital for sustainable social and behavioral change. In the current resource-scarce reality of BRs, however, the approach that requires community initiation for projects also limits most activities to the topics of community partner interests.

The perceived mandates of both stakeholders and the bridging organizations appear to influence cross-sectoral collaboration in a much more complex manner than anticipated. The BR organizations that did not explicitly integrate health into their activities did not see health as part of their mandate, whereas those focusing on health did interpret the same UNESCO mandate as inherently including health. Evidently some ambiguity surrounds the term 'well-being' and whether it is about health or sustainable development. While health stakeholders see health and well-being as synonymous, other influential voices, for instance the Government of Wales, treat well-being as identical to sustainable development. This vagueness of terms can facilitate cross-sectoral collaboration, but it also may cause unnecessary variation in interpretation of the mandates.

Similarly, interpretations of the institutional mandates were important factors determining the ability of local health professionals to engage actively in BR activities. Responses indicated that frontline health practitioners often feel strictly limited by their narrow mandates, despite the personal perceptions of the relevance of cross-sectoral integrated approach to health promotion. Particularly, environmental health practitioners are often excluded from professional collaborations, because their heavy workload is strictly guided by government directives. This is precisely the problem that Rittel and Webber identified in 1973 (19), when they developed the concept of "wicked problems".

The perceptions of upper management within healthcare organizations also strongly influence how government dictated mandates are understood and to which extent innovative cross-sectoral collaboration is encouraged in practice. For instance, in Ontario, some health units are engaged with their local BRs, whereas others remain unresponsive to invitations. Moreover, some participants expressed a desire to engage primary health care providers, e.g. to issue Green Gym prescriptions (promoting outdoors activities instead of prescription drugs or inside gyms) or to discuss the potential role of nature in mental health therapy. These findings suggest that the health sector might benefit from a more open approach to stakeholder engagement. Indeed, broad cross-sectoral engagement of unconventional partners is encouraged particularly by the settings-based health promotion perspective (29).

All participants throughout the study recognized that they had limited knowledge and understanding of one another's mandates. This was evident whether or not any active cross-sectoral collaboration with the health stakeholders was taking place. The admitted ignorance illustrates how personal perceptions, interpersonal interaction, and sense of mutual trust appears to play a much greater role in the initiation of collaborative activities than actual shared knowledge. Trust has been identified as a key factor in cross-sectoral collaboration (30), but it would be interesting to explore the impact of better mutual understanding of the mandates of respective partners on potential partnership development. The lack of knowledge about others' mandates does not necessarily prevent cooperation, as long as an overall understanding of shared issues is present. It, however, appeared to cause some form of a barrier to people's ability to identify potential unconventional collaborators.

An explicit, open, cross-sectoral dialogue might enhance the integration of health and sustainable development. The potential for more extensive bridging activities was exemplified by one environmental stakeholder, who stated that: "To be totally honest, until quite recently, I haven't given the relationship with human health a great deal of thought. But when I think about it, it is actually extremely relevant, even though the management is focused on the ecosystem and habitat and species. It is actually extremely important for human health as well, because of things like water storage, carbon storage, and the other ecosystem services that the site provides". Similarly, the public health management attendance at a meeting on integrated community sustainability plans, organized by the local BR, resulted the following statement: "It was an exciting meeting and really helped me see how our work in public health fits within the sustainable community's movement".

A number of participating non-health stakeholders pointed out that many current limitations to health-related activities reflect limited understanding of possible public health matters. In general, biosphere participants recognized that the focus of activities within their respective organizations is usually directly dependent on the engaged individuals and their expertise or interests. Only where health professionals are actively participating does health promotion become an explicit component of the bridging efforts. As noted above, open cross-sectoral discussions contain the potential to stimulate action. For example, one Canadian BR was recently inspired to partner with the local health unit to arrange walking groups and invited the engaged Public Health Nurse to join their Board.

While BRs are effective bridging organizations bringing diverse stakeholders together (see table 2), interviewees reported that it was a challenge finding the right language to attract the health sector to join meetings. Forty years after the globally recognized Lalonde Report (31) declared environment as a determinant of health, the health sector evidently remains slow to engage with environmental stakeholders. The interview results reveal that integrating health in projects outside the health sector still depends directly on individuals who take it upon themselves to bring people together. Although each BR organization clearly is driven by a group of passionate people, the current success of health stakeholder integration seems to depend on a few visionary individuals, who are good at connecting people. Some of these community champions work within the health sector and others are networkers within BR organizations who see health as an integral component of sustainable communities. Studies on effectiveness of community-based health promotion support the value of community champions in driving change (32).

Despite the barriers, BRs have had some success in developing cross-sectoral activities that promote health-related changes both at the individual behavior and the systems level (see table 2). Not all interviewees saw the necessity of having an explicit focus on health in BRs' program development. As one participant pointed out: "I think [health] is implicit in what we're doing already." To justify the shift to explicit health focus would require, for instance, availability of some health funding consistent with the criteria set for BR activities. That said, making the implicit explicit would probably also help health practitioners justify their participation in cross-sectoral collaboration with BRs.

This study indicates that organizations with primary focus other than health have a potential to play a meaningful role in providing a neutral, apolitical, platform that helps bringing diverse community stakeholders to the table to promote health. In the case of BRs, this potential could be significantly increased by making health an explicit part of the BR mandate and exploring the mandates of potential health-related partners in greater detail. The health sector within BR regions, in turn, has an innovative opportunity not only to promote health but also to facilitate application of 'Health in All Policies' approach. In addition to ideological goals, such collaboration could strengthen the local health promotion capacity in resource-strapped rural communities. This would, however, require more proactive strategies among the health professionals. In general, BRs have a great potential role as bridging organizations that help integrate health and sustainable development in practice. The in-depth qualitative analysis reported here indicates that this type of bridging organization represents a promising new venue for meaningful solutions to wicked public health problems at the community-level.

Acknowledgments

This research was partially funded by the Canadian Social Sciences and Humanities Research Council (SSHRC).

References

[1] World Health Organization (WHO) Bangkok Charter for Health Promotion. URL: http://www.who.int/healthpromotion/conferences/6gchp/bangkok_charter/en/

[2] WHO, Government of South Australia. The Adelaide Statement on Health in All Policies: moving towards a shared governance for health and well-being. Health Promot Int 2010;25:258-60.

[3] Born P. Creating vibrant communities: How individuals and organizations from diverse sectors of society are coming together to reduce poverty in Canada. Toronto: BPS Books, 2010.

[4] Harting J, Kunst AE, Kwan A, Stronks K. A 'health broker' role as a catalyst of change to promote health: An experiment in deprived Dutch neighbourhoods. Health Promot Int 2011;26(1):65-81.

[5] UNESCO [homepage on the Internet]. What is a biosphere reserve? Paris: UNESCO Headquarters, 2014. URL: www.unesco.org/mab/doc/faq/brs.pdf.

[6] UNESCO [homepage on the Internet]. Biosphere Reserves – Learning Sites for Sustainable Development. Paris: UNESCO Headquarters, 2014. URL: http://www.unesco.org/

[7] Francis G. Biosphere reserves in Canada: Ideals and some experience. Environ 2004;32(3):3-26.

[8] Nguyen NC, Bosch OJ, Maani KE. Creating 'learning laboratories' for sustainable development in biospheres: A systems thinking approach. Syst Res Behav Sci 2011;28(1):51-62.

[9] Matysek KA, Stratford E, Kriwoken LK. The UNESCO biosphere reserve program in Australia: Constraints and opportunities for localized sustainable development. Can Geogr 2006;50(1):85-100.
[10] Brown LD. Bridging organizations and sustainable development. Hum Relat 1991;44(8):807-31.
[11] Schultz L. Nurturing resilience in social-ecological systems: Lessons learned from bridging organizations. Dissertation. Stockholm: Stockholm University, 2009.
[12] Biggs R, Westley FR, Carpenter SR. Navigating the back loop: Fostering social innovation and transformation in ecosystem management. Ecol Soc 2010;15(2):28.
[13] Crona BI, Parker JN. Learning in support of governance: Theories, methods, and a framework to assess how bridging organizations contribute to adaptive resource governance. Ecol Soc 2012;17(1):32.
[14] Malayang BSI, Hahn T, Kumar P. Responses to ecosystem change and to their impacts on human well-being. Millennium ecosystem assessment, ecosystems and human well-being: Multiscale assessments: Findings of the sub-global assessments working group. Washington, DC: Island Press, 2007: 203-28.
[15] Berkes F. Devolution of environment and resources governance: Trends and future. Environ Conserv 2010;37(4):489-500.
[16] Hahn T, Olsson P, Folke C, Johansson K. Trust-building, knowledge generation and organizational innovations: The role of a bridging organization for adaptive comanagement of a wetland landscape around Kristianstad, Sweden. Hum Ecol 2006;34:573-92.
[17] Berkes F. Evolution of co-management: Role of knowledge generation, bridging organizations and social learning. J Environ Manage 2009;90(5):1692-1702.
[18] Schultz L, Duit A, Folke C. Participation, adaptive co-management, and management performance in the world network of biosphere reserves. World Dev 2011;39(4):662-71.
[19] Rittel HWJ, Webber MM. Dilemmas in a general theory of planning. Policy Sci 1973;4(2):155-69.
[20] Kreuter MW, De Rosa C, Howze EH, Baldwin GT. Understanding wicked problems: A key to advancing environmental health promotion. Health Educ Behav 2004;31(4):441-54.
[21] Caron RM, Serrell N. Community ecology and capacity: Keys to progressing the environmental communication of wicked problems. Appl Environ Educ Commun 2009;8(3-4):195-203.
[22] Brown V, Harris J, Russell J. Tackling wicked problems through the transdisciplinary imagination. London: Earthscan, 2010.
[23] Patton MQ. Qualitative research and evaluation methods. Thousand Oaks, CA: Sage, 2002.
[24] UNESCO [homepage on the internet]. Madrid Action Plan. Paris: UNESCO Headquarters, 2014. URL: http://www.unesco.org/
[25] Nutbeam D, Harris E. Theory in a nutshell: a practical guide to health promotion theories. Sydney: McGraw-Hill Australia, 2004.
[26] Bartholomew LK, Parcel GS, Kok G, Gottlieb NH editors. Planning health promotion programs: an intervention mapping approach. San Francisco, CA: Jossey-Bass, 2006.
[27] Minkler M editor. Community organizing and community building for health. New Brunswick, NJ: Rutgers University Press, 1997.
[28] Kretzmann JP, McKnight J. Building communities from the inside out: a path toward finding and mobilizing a community's assets. Evanston, IL: Asset-Based Community Development Institute, Institute Policy Research, Northwestern University, 1993.
[29] Poland BD, Green L, Rootman I. Settings for health promotion: Linking theory and practice. London: Sage, 2000:1–43.
[30] Wakefield SEL, Poland BD. Family, friend or foe? Critical reflections on the relevance and role of social capital in health promotion and community development. Soc Sci Med 2005;60(12):2819-32.
[31] Health Canada. Lalonde Report: A new perspective on the health of Canadians: a working document. Ottawa, ON: Health Canada, 1974.
[32] Popay J, Attree P, Hornby D, Milton B, Whitehead M, French B, et al. Community engagement in initiatives addressing the wider social determinants of health: A rapid review of evidence on impact, experience and process. Soc Determinants Effectiveness Rev 2007:1-226. URL: www.nice.org.uk/nicemedia/live/11929/44494/44494.pdf

Section four: Acknowledgments

In: Public Health
Editors: Rosemary M. Caron and Joav Merrick
ISBN: 978-1-63321-569-6

Chapter 17

About the editors

Rosemary M Caron, PhD, MPH is an associate professor, Director of Undergraduate Studies, and the former Director of the Master of Public Health Program in the Department of Health Management and Policy, College of Health and Human Services; Core Faculty in the New Hampshire Leadership Education in Neurodevelopmental Disabilities; Fellow in the Carsey Institue; and Adjunct Associate Professor in the Master's of Community Development Policy and Practice Program, Graduate School at the University of New Hampshire, Durham, New Hampshire, United States of America. Dr. Caron is also an Adjunct Associate Professor of Pediatrics in the Department of Pediatrics at the Geisel School of Medicine in Hanover, New Hampshire, United States of America. Dr. Caron teaches undergraduate and graduate students in public health and healthcare management. She received the "2011 Teaching Excellence Award" from the College of Health and Human Services. Her research interests and publications reflect the multi-disciplinary nature of public health and are based on professional and academic experiences in building community capacity to address persistent public health issues; and improving and expanding public health education at the undergraduate and graduate levels in the healthcare management curriculum and related disciplines. Prior research funding addressed developing and integrating effective pedagogy of public health courses into the undergraduate curriculum at liberal arts institutions and community technical colleges. Prior to entering academia, Dr. Caron practiced public health for several years in a variety of settings as a practitioner. Specifically, she worked as the Assistant State Epidemiologist in the Bureau of Health Risk Assessment and she served as the Chief of the Bureau of Health Statistics and Data Management for the New Hampshire Department of Health and Human Services, New Hampshire, USA. At New Hampshire's largest local health department, she worked as a Chronic Disease Epidemiologist and Environmental Toxicologist. Dr. Caron is a current member of the American Public Health Association (APHA) and has regularly presented her research at the annual APHA meetings. She participates in the Public Health Education and Health Promotion and Community Health Policy Development Sections of APHA. She is a former member of the Board of Directors for the New Hampshire Public Health Association, the state affiliate of the APHA. She is a current member of the Association of University Programs in Health Administration and is the former Chair of the Public Health Faculty Network for this organization. She is also a current member of the Board of Directors of the American College of Epidemiology and the

Association of Prevention, Teaching and Research. She is also a current member of the National Environmental Health Association and the American College of Healthcare Executives. She is an Associate Editor for the Association of Prevention, Teaching and Research Prevention Education Resource Center and the Public Health Education and Promotion Section of Frontiers. Dr. Caron has numerous peer-reviewed journal publications, book chapters, and editorials to her credit. She has edited several books, authored one book on the public health workforce, and is in the process of authoring a textbook on population health management. She also serves as a peer reviewer for nationally and internationally-renowned journals and is on the Editorial Board of several prominent journals. E-mail: Rosemary.Caron@unh.edu

Joav Merrick, MD, MMedSci, DMSc, is professor of pediatrics, child health and human development, Division of Pediatrics, Hadassah Hebrew University Medical Center, Mt Scopus Campus, Jerusalem, Israel and Kentucky Children's Hospital, University of Kentucky, Lexington, Kentucky United States and professor of public health at the Center for Healthy Development, School of Public Health, Georgia State University, Atlanta, United States, the medical director of the Health Services, Division for Intellectual and Developmental Disabilities, Ministry of Social Affairs and Social Services, Jerusalem, the founder and director of the National Institute of Child Health and Human Development in Israel. Numerous publications in the field of pediatrics, child health and human development, rehabilitation, intellectual disability, disability, health, welfare, abuse, advocacy, quality of life and prevention. Received the Peter Sabroe Child Award for outstanding work on behalf of Danish Children in 1985 and the International LEGO-Prize ("The Children's Nobel Prize") for an extraordinary contribution towards improvement in child welfare and well-being in 1987. E-mail: jmerrick@zahav.net.il

In: Public Health
Editors: Rosemary M. Caron and Joav Merrick
ISBN: 978-1-63321-569-6

Chapter 18

About the Department of Health Management and Policy, College of Health and Human Services, University of New Hampshire, USA

The University of New Hampshire, located in Durham, New Hampshire, USA is part of the University System of New Hampshire. The Health Management and Policy (HMP) Department, which began in 1975, is housed in the College of Health and Human Services and offers a Bachelor of Science (B.S.) degree in HMP. In 2007, the HMP Department established a track in the undergraduate major that permits students to elect a series of public health courses offered through the Department. In addition, for several years, the Department has offered all UNH students the opportunity to complete a five course minor in public health.

The HMP Department is comprised of tenured, tenure-track, research, clinical, and adjunct faculty who possess a wide breadth of knowledge and practical experience in public health and health care. We have a well-established curriculum that offers courses in health management and policy and public health. The HMP faculty are also engaged in research projects that examine population health, public health education, health care and financial systems, health policy and program evaluation.

In addition to an established undergraduate curriculum, the HMP Department administers the UNH Master of Public Health (MPH) Program, a general MPH Program that began in 2001 and was initially accredited by the Council on Education in Public Health in 2005. The MPH Program is designed for working professionals from a wide variety of professional backgrounds.

UNH Department of Health Management and Policy website: http://www.chhs.unh.edu/hmp/undergradhmp_program.html

Contact

Associate Professor Rosemary M Caron, PhD, MPH
University of New Hampshire
College of Health and Human Services
Department of Health Management and Policy

319 Hewitt Hall, 4 Library Way
Durham, New Hampshire 03824
United States of America
E-mail: Rosemary.Caron@unh.edu

In: Public Health
Editors: Rosemary M. Caron and Joav Merrick
ISBN: 978-1-63321-569-6

Chapter 19

About the National Institute of Child Health and Human Development in Israel

The National Institute of Child Health and Human Development (NICHD) in Israel was established in 1998 as a virtual institute under the auspicies of the Medical Director, Ministry of Social Affairs and Social Services in order to function as the research arm for the Office of the Medical Director. In 1998 the National Council for Child Health and Pediatrics, Ministry of Health and in 1999 the Director General and Deputy Director General of the Ministry of Health endorsed the establishment of the NICHD.

Mission

The mission of a National Institute for Child Health and Human Development in Israel is to provide an academic focal point for the scholarly interdisciplinary study of child life, health, public health, welfare, disability, rehabilitation, intellectual disability and related aspects of human development. This mission includes research, teaching, clinical work, information and public service activities in the field of child health and human development.

Service and academic activities

Over the years many activities became focused in the south of Israel due to collaboration with various professionals at the Faculty of Health Sciences (FOHS) at the Ben Gurion University of the Negev (BGU). Since 2000 an affiliation with the Zusman Child Development Center at the Pediatric Division of Soroka University Medical Center has resulted in collaboration around the establishment of the Down Syndrome Clinic at that center. In 2002 a full course on "Disability" was established at the Recanati School for Allied Professions in the Community, FOHS, BGU and in 2005 collaboration was started with the Primary Care Unit of the faculty and disability became part of the master of public health course on "Children and society". In the academic year 2005-2006 a one semester course on "Aging with disability" was started as part of the master of science program in gerontology in our collaboration with the Center for Multidisciplinary Research in Aging. In 2010 collaborations with the Division of Pediatrics, Hadassah Hebrew University Medical Center, Jerusalem, Israel around the National Down Syndrome Center and teaching students and residents about intellectual and developmental disabilities as part of their training at this campus.

Research activities

The affiliated staff have over the years published work from projects and research activities in this national and international collaboration. In the year 2000 the International Journal of Adolescent Medicine and Health and in 2005 the International Journal on Disability and Human Development of De Gruyter Publishing House (Berlin and New York) were affiliated with the National Institute of Child Health and Human Development. From 2008 also the International Journal of Child Health and Human Development (Nova Science, New York), the International Journal of Child and Adolescent Health (Nova Science) and the Journal of Pain Management (Nova Science) affiliated and from 2009 the International Public Health Journal (Nova Science) and Journal of Alternative Medicine Research (Nova Science). All peer-reviewed international journals.

National collaborations

Nationally the NICHD works in collaboration with the Faculty of Health Sciences, Ben Gurion University of the Negev; Department of Physical Therapy, Sackler School of Medicine, Tel Aviv University; Autism Center, Assaf HaRofeh Medical Center; National Rett and PKU Centers at Chaim Sheba Medical Center, Tel HaShomer; Department of Physiotherapy, Haifa University; Department of Education, Bar Ilan University, Ramat Gan, Faculty of Social Sciences and Health Sciences; College of Judea and Samaria in Ariel and in 2011 affiliation with Center for Pediatric Chronic Diseases and National Center for Down Syndrome, Department of Pediatrics, Hadassah Hebrew University Medical Center, Mount Scopus Campus, Jerusalem.

International collaborations

Internationally with the Department of Disability and Human Development, College of Applied Health Sciences, University of Illinois at Chicago; Strong Center for Developmental Disabilities, Golisano Children's Hospital at Strong, University of Rochester School of Medicine and Dentistry, New York; Centre on Intellectual Disabilities, University of Albany, New York; Centre for Chronic Disease Prevention and Control, Health Canada, Ottawa; Chandler Medical Center and Children's Hospital, Kentucky Children's Hospital, Section of Adolescent Medicine, University of Kentucky, Lexington; Chronic Disease Prevention and Control Research Center, Baylor College of Medicine, Houston, Texas; Division of Neuroscience, Department of Psychiatry, Columbia University, New York; Institute for the Study of Disadvantage and Disability, Atlanta; Center for Autism and Related Disorders,

Department Psychiatry, Children's Hospital Boston, Boston; Department of Paediatrics, Child Health and Adolescent Medicine, Children's Hospital at Westmead, Westmead, Australia; International Centre for the Study of Occupational and Mental Health, Düsseldorf, Germany; Centre for Advanced Studies in Nursing, Department of General Practice and Primary Care, University of Aberdeen, Aberdeen, United Kingdom; Quality of Life Research Center, Copenhagen, Denmark; Nordic School of Public Health, Gottenburg, Sweden, Scandinavian Institute of Quality of Working Life, Oslo, Norway; The Department of Applied Social Sciences (APSS) of The Hong Kong Polytechnic University Hong Kong.

Targets

Our focus is on research, international collaborations, clinical work, teaching and policy in health, disability and human development and to establish the NICHD as a permanent institute at one of the residential care centers for persons with intellectual disability in Israel in order to conduct model research and together with the four university schools of public health/medicine in Israel establish a national master and doctoral program in disability and human development at the institute to secure the next generation of professionals working in this often non-prestigious/low-status field of work.

Contact

Joav Merrick, MD, MMedSci, DMSc
Professor of Pediatrics, Child Health and Human Development
Medical Director, Health Services,
Division for Intellectual and Developmental Disabilities,
Ministry of Social Affairs and Social Services, POB 1260, IL-91012 Jerusalem, Israel.
E-mail: jmerrick@zahav.net.il

ISBN: 978-1-63321-569-6

Chapter 20

About the book series "Health and Human Development"

Health and human development is a book series with publications from a multidisciplinary group of researchers, practitioners and clinicians for an international professional forum interested in the broad spectrum of health and human development. Books already published:

- Merrick J, Omar HA, eds. Adolescent behavior research. International perspectives. New York: Nova Science, 2007.
- Kratky KW. Complementary medicine systems: Comparison and integration. New York: Nova Science, 2008.
- Schofield P, Merrick J, eds. Pain in children and youth. New York: Nova Science, 2009.
- Greydanus DE, Patel DR, Pratt HD, Calles Jr JL, eds. Behavioral pediatrics, 3 ed. New York: Nova Science, 2009.
- Ventegodt S, Merrick J, eds. Meaningful work: Research in quality of working life. New York: Nova Science, 2009.
- Omar HA, Greydanus DE, Patel DR, Merrick J, eds. Obesity and adolescence. A public health concern. New York: Nova Science, 2009.
- Lieberman A, Merrick J, eds. Poverty and children. A public health concern. New York: Nova Science, 2009.
- Goodbread J. Living on the edge. The mythical, spiritual and philosophical roots of social marginality. New York: Nova Science, 2009.
- Bennett DL, Towns S, Elliot E, Merrick J, eds. Challenges in adolescent health: An Australian perspective. New York: Nova Science, 2009.
- Schofield P, Merrick J, eds. Children and pain. New York: Nova Science, 2009.
- Sher L, Kandel I, Merrick J, eds. Alcohol-related cognitive disorders: Research and clinical perspectives. New York: Nova Science, 2009.
- Anyanwu EC. Advances in environmental health effects of toxigenic mold and mycotoxins. New York: Nova Science, 2009.
- Bell E, Merrick J, eds. Rural child health. International aspects. New York: Nova Science, 2009.
- Dubowitz H, Merrick J, eds. International aspects of child abuse and neglect. New York: Nova Science, 2010.

- Shahtahmasebi S, Berridge D. Conceptualizing behavior: A practical guide to data analysis. New York: Nova Science, 2010.
- Wernik U. Chance action and therapy. The playful way of changing. New York: Nova Science, 2010.
- Omar HA, Greydanus DE, Patel DR, Merrick J, eds. Adolescence and chronic illness. A public health concern. New York: Nova Science, 2010.
- Patel DR, Greydanus DE, Omar HA, Merrick J, eds. Adolescence and sports. New York: Nova Science, 2010.
- Shek DTL, Ma HK, Merrick J, eds. Positive youth development: Evaluation and future directions in a Chinese context. New York: Nova Science, 2010.
- Shek DTL, Ma HK, Merrick J, eds. Positive youth development: Implementation of a youth program in a Chinese context. New York: Nova Science, 2010.
- Omar HA, Greydanus DE, Tsitsika AK, Patel DR, Merrick J, eds. Pediatric and adolescent sexuality and gynecology: Principles for the primary care clinician. New York: Nova Science, 2010.
- Chow E, Merrick J, eds. Advanced cancer. Pain and quality of life. New York: Nova Science, 2010.
- Latzer Y, Merrick, J, Stein D, eds. Understanding eating disorders. Integrating culture, psychology and biology. New York: Nova Science, 2010.
- Sahgal A, Chow E, Merrick J, eds. Bone and brain metastases: Advances in research and treatment. New York: Nova Science, 2010.
- Postolache TT, Merrick J, eds. Environment, mood disorders and suicide. New York: Nova Science, 2010.
- Maharajh HD, Merrick J, eds. Social and cultural psychiatry experience from the Caribbean Region. New York: Nova Science, 2010.
- Mirsky J. Narratives and meanings of migration. New York: Nova Science, 2010.
- Harvey PW. Self-management and the health care consumer. New York: Nova Science, 2011.
- Ventegodt S, Merrick J. Sexology from a holistic point of view. New York: Nova Science, 2011.
- Ventegodt S, Merrick J. Principles of holistic psychiatry: A textbook on holistic medicine for mental disorders. New York: Nova Science, 2011.
- Greydanus DE, Calles Jr JL, Patel DR, Nazeer A, Merrick J, eds. Clinical aspects of psychopharmacology in childhood and adolescence. New York: Nova Science, 2011.
- Bell E, Seidel BM, Merrick J, eds. Climate change and rural child health. New York: Nova Science, 2011.
- Bell E, Zimitat C, Merrick J, eds. Rural medical education: Practical strategies. New York: Nova Science, 2011.
- Latzer Y, Tzischinsky. The dance of sleeping and eating among adolescents: Normal and pathological perspectives. New York: Nova Science, 2011.
- Deshmukh VD. The astonishing brain and holistic consciousness: Neuroscience and Vedanta perspectives. New York: Nova Science, 2011.
- Bell E, Westert GP, Merrick J, eds. Translational research for primary healthcare. New York: Nova Science, 2011.
- Shek DTL, Sun RCF, Merrick J, eds. Drug abuse in Hong Kong: Development and evaluation of a prevention program. New York: Nova Science, 2011.
- Ventegodt S, Hermansen TD, Merrick J. Human Development: Biology from a holistic point of view. New York: Nova Science, 2011.

- Ventegodt S, Merrick J. Our search for meaning in life. New York: Nova Science, 2011.
- Caron RM, Merrick J, eds. Building community capacity: Minority and immigrant populations. New York: Nova Science, 2012.
- Klein H, Merrick J, eds. Human immunodeficiency virus (HIV) research: Social science aspects. New York: Nova Science, 2012.
- Lutzker JR, Merrick J, eds. Applied public health: Examining multifaceted Social or ecological problems and child maltreatment. New York: Nova Science, 2012.
- Chemtob D, Merrick J, eds. AIDS and tuberculosis: Public health aspects. New York: Nova Science, 2012.
- Ventegodt S, Merrick J. Textbook on evidence-based holistic mind-body medicine: Basic principles of healing in traditional Hippocratic medicine. New York: Nova Science, 2012.
- Ventegodt S, Merrick J. Textbook on evidence-based holistic mind-body medicine: Holistic practice of traditional Hippocratic medicine. New York: Nova Science, 2012.
- Ventegodt S, Merrick J. Textbook on evidence-based holistic mind-body medicine: Healing the mind in traditional Hippocratic medicine. New York: Nova Science, 2012.
- Ventegodt S, Merrick J. Textbook on evidence-based holistic mind-body medicine: Sexology and traditional Hippocratic medicine. New York: Nova Science, 2012.
- Ventegodt S, Merrick J. Textbook on evidence-based holistic mind-body medicine: Research, philosophy, economy and politics of traditional Hippocratic medicine. New York: Nova Science, 2012.
- Caron RM, Merrick J, eds. Building community capacity: Skills and principles. New York: Nova Science, 2012.
- Lemal M, Merrick J, eds. Health risk communication. New York: Nova Science, 2012.
- Ventegodt S, Merrick J. Textbook on evidence-based holistic mind-body medicine: Basic philosophy and ethics of traditional Hippocratic medicine. New York: Nova Science, 2013.
- Caron RM, Merrick J, eds. Building community capacity: Case examples from around the world. New York: Nova Science, 2013.
- Steele RE. Managed care in a public setting. New York: Nova Science, 2013.
- Srabstein JC, Merrick J, eds. Bullying: A public health concern. New York: Nova Science, 2013.
- Pulenzas N, Lechner B, Thavarajah N, Chow E, Merrick J, eds. Advanced cancer: Managing symptoms and quality of life. New York: Nova Science, 2013.
- Stein D, Latzer Y, eds. Treatment and recovery of eating disorders. New York: Nova Science, 2013.
- Sun J, Buys N, Merrick J. Health promotion: Community singing as a vehicle to promote health. New York: Nova Science, 2013.
- Pulenzas N, Lechner B, Thavarajah N, Chow E, Merrick J, eds. Advanced cancer: Managing symptoms and quality of life. New York: Nova Science, 2013.
- Sun J, Buys N, Merrick J. Health promotion: Strengthening positive health and preventing disease. New York: Nova Science, 2013.
- Merrick J, Israeli S, eds. Food, nutrition and eating behavior. New York: Nova Science, 2013.
- Shahtahmasebi S, Merrick J. Suicide from a public health perspective.

- New York: Nova Science, 2014.
- Merrick J, Tenenbaum A, eds. Public health concern: Smoking, alcohol and substance use. New York: Nova Science, 2014.
- Merrick J, Aspler S, Morad M, eds. Mental health from an international perspective. New York: Nova Science, 2014.
- Merrick J, ed. India: Health and human development aspects. New York: Nova Science, 2014.

Contact

Professor Joav Merrick, MD, MMedSci, DMSc
Medical Director, Health Services
Division for Intellectual and Developmental Disabailities
Ministry of Social Affairs and Social Services
POBox 1260, IL-91012 Jerusalem, Israel
E-mail: jmerrick@zahav.net.il

Section five: Index

Index

B

C

D

E

F

G

H

I

J

K

L

M

Q

R

S

T

U

V

W

Y